THE HAPPIEST DIET IN THE WORLD

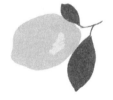

THE HAPPIEST DIET IN THE WORLD

How to eat like the healthiest people on earth

GIULIA CROUCH

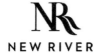

NEW RIVER

Disclaimer

The material in this book is for informational purposes only. As each individual situation is unique, you should use proper discretion, in consultation with a health care practitioner, before undertaking the diet and techniques described in this book. The author and publisher expressly disclaim responsibility for any adverse effects that may result from the use or application of the information it contains.

Published in 2024 by New River Books
www.newriverbooks.co.uk

10 9 8 7 6 5 4 3 2 1

Copyright © Giulia Crouch 2024

Giulia Crouch has asserted her right under the Copyright, Designs and Patents Act 1988 to be identified as the author of this work. All rights reserved. No part of this publication may be reproduced, stored in a retrieval system or transmitted in any form, or by any means (electronic, mechanical, or otherwise) without the prior written permission of both the copyright owners and the publisher.

A CIP catalogue record for this book is available from the British Library.

ISBN: 978-1-915780-14-0

Recipe consultant: Kathryn Bruton
Photography: Smith & Gilmour
Cover design and illustrations: Jo Walker

Printed and bound in the UK by CPI.

This FSC label means that materials used for the product have been responsibly sourced.

*To dad, for reading my childhood "novels"
and teaching me how to think about writing.*

Roger Stephen Crouch 1956 - 2011

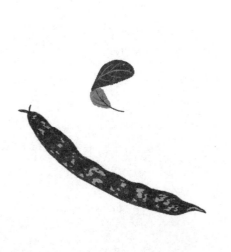

CONTENTS

Introduction   9

1 The way we eat in The West   23
Hayley's fridge
The Western paradox
Are you enjoying that?

2 The diet of the blue zones   42
Carbs are not the enemy
Powerful plants
Meat as seasoning
Legumes for life
Daily nuts
Liquid gold
What's the deal with dairy?
Deliberate sugar
The curious role of wine

3 Old wisdom, new science   99
Fasting and longevity
Magical food combinations
Why counting calories is a waste of time
The complete absence of UPFs
Gut feelings
The psychology of eating together
Nutritional intelligence
Food at the heart of a nourishing lifestyle

4 Five steps to a happier diet   145

Recipes   165

Endnotes, Index

Introduction

As a food writer, I'm often invited to hot restaurants serving cool food; rich, elaborate and exquisitely plated dishes with difficult-to-source ingredients; tiny, precise garnishes and flamboyant foams. And yet when someone asks me, which they often do, what my all-time favourite dish is, or what I'd choose as my last meal on earth, the same answer always cartwheels to mind: my nonna's tomato pasta.

People tend to be disappointed by this, so I quickly come up with something else. My Italian grandmother would always make a lightly dressed green salad as a second course, I tell them, which I'd certainly have on my dream menu as well!

"*Seriou*sly?" my quizzer will say. "A *food* writer, who's eaten in the most sought-after, hard-to-get-a-table-at restaurants in this vast and rich culinary mecca we call London, only wants *pasta in tomato sauce* and *green salad?*"

I know why they're dissatisfied. They expect my choice to be outlandish, decadent or intricate; to reflect the character of the amazing dishes I've eaten prepared by some of the country's best chefs. They're primed to hear words like *lobster*, *truffle*, *brown butter* and *bisque* or for me to talk about complicated cooking techniques involving expensive kit and professional skills honed over years. They don't want to be presented with a basic peasant dish of tomato, flour and water.

It sounds plain, boring, bland even. But it wasn't. It was

perfect; an irreproachable example of the brilliance that occurs when you combine minimal ingredients with a cook's wisdom. In simplicity it is easier to create surprise. I remember the dish so well I can almost smell it.

My grandmother, Vincenzina Marzio (called Enza for short in the UK), was born in the south of Italy in 1931, in a village 50km north of Naples in Campania, a region known for the creation of pizza and the dramatic beauty of its Amalfi Coast. Nonna's village is not by the sea, however, but inland; a small, rural place that's given a sense of vastness and peace by the two mountains that loom calmly over it, like two friendly bodyguards on shift.

In the 1950s, Nonna moved to England, where she met my grandfather, a Sardinian who'd also upped sticks after the war for Blighty. Together, they had four children – one of whom was my mother, Paola. After living in the Midlands for a few years, the family decided to move further south, to Kent, as it was just too cold "up north". It is there, in their small, terraced house, with gardens at the front and back (where they grew cucumbers, peas, figs and potatoes), that we find my nonna's table. On it is a large glass bowl filled with bouncy coils of fusilli, each one coated in a slick, silken, orangey-red sauce.

The air in the room smelt sweet and I still remember the squelch of the metal spoon as Nonna dug it into the bowl. We'd go crazy for cheese, so finely grated it was like freshly fallen powder snow. It was often put in a sugar shaker for ease; something that would cause me much confusion and one sugary dinner, at a pizzeria later in life. And then, we ate.

A wonderful alchemy happens when you cook tomatoes, resulting in a flavour combination that is sweet, acidic and savoury all at once – and elevated further by the fatty, salty richness of the Parmesan. Sometimes, idly gazing into the bowl, I'd spot a wilted plume of parsley stuck to the side. It wasn't for eating but instead worked like a teabag, infusing the sauce with its subtle flavour and aroma. You wouldn't think a small bunch of herbs could make such a difference to the final result, but it did, and now parsley cooked in a tomato sauce – though I don't often encounter it outside my mum's cooking – is the smell I most associate with my nonna. It was the signature motif of her cuisine.

Ever since then, there's been a special place in my heart for this style of cooking; the quietly masterful kind that can take nothing much and turn it into something dazzling. As many genius things do, it came from necessity. Where my nonna came from they didn't have a lot, so they made the best of what they did have, and learnt, through trial and error and shared wisdom, to achieve deliciousness. Meat was expensive or unavailable so didn't feature much in their cooking, and when it did, it was used sparingly; treated more like a way to season other food than the point of focus. Or was celebrated with fanfare – a whole roasted pig for a festival or other special occasion. In its place were all sorts of plants. Abundant vegetables of the region included tomatoes, aubergines and dark leafy greens. My grandmother loved them – the more bitter the better – wilted down with olive oil and garlic. In fact, the whole region developed such a taste for these greens that the rest of Italy took to calling them *mangiafoglie* or "leaf-eaters".

Beans were very important, a cheap staple, which through loving respect and care were made to taste amazing. *Pasta e fagioli* (pasta and beans), *zuppa di fagioli e patate* (bean and potato soup), *cicoria e fagioli* (leafy greens and beans) and even a savoury bean and stale bread pudding cooked in the oven until soft and deliciously comforting.

A starter (fermented flour and water that acts as a leavening agent in traditional baking) for bread was shared from house to house and after it was cooked, they'd use the heat from the outdoor oven to roast artichokes and peppers. Vegetables were preserved *sott'olio* so that they could be eaten later in the year, but otherwise the menu was dictated by the season. Winter meant artichokes and cauliflower; spring, peas and zucchini flowers; summer, tomatoes, peppers and aubergine; and autumn, porcini mushrooms and chestnuts.

Frugality is the mother of invention. *Panzanella*, a bread salad with tomato and lashings of olive oil, now a fashionable starter in certain chic restaurants, was created as a way to use up stale odds and ends. *Cacio e pepe* is pasta in nothing but cheese and pepper, and yet in recent times this extremely basic dish whipped everyone up into a frenzy of adoration with queues around the block.

Nonna continued to cook these kinds of things after moving to England and now it's the food I love and crave the most.

It's not just in rural Italy that cuisine is guided by seasonality and frugality. Ratatouille, a sweet stew of aubergines, peppers and courgette, was invented by French farmers as a way of using up summer vegetables, and *khichdi*, an Indian dish of just rice and lentils cooked with spices and tempered with ghee, is the humblest of recipes but also one of the nation's favourites. In the Balkans, they love *pasulj*, a simple but soul-warming bean soup made with very few ingredients, that leaves you marvelling at how wonderful beans are.

Why am I telling you this? Well, because it turns out this kind of cooking, the traditional cooking of my grandparents, and that of many other communities around the world, may possess a secret we could all do with knowing.

The blue zones

There are places around the world where people live for an unusually long time compared to the rest of us. They're called the *blue zones*. This may prompt pictures of azure skies or sapphire seas, but the etymology is, sadly, less romantic. They were so called after the colour of the felt-tip pen used by the scientist who was pinpointing the area on a map of Sardinia, Italy's second-largest island after Sicily and the home of my grandfather. Sardinia is a rugged and captivating land with a distinct identity, set apart from the mainland via language (they speak Sardinian, not Italian) and culture.

Dr Gianni Pes, a senior researcher in the Department of Clinical and Experimental Medicine at the University of Sassari, in the north of the island, was the scientist with the blue pen. He began studying longevity in the 1990s, after being inspired by his great-uncle, Pasquale Frasconi, who, having lived to age 110, was not just a centenarian but a *supercentenarian*. Another of his relatives had made it to 97, which though 13 years shy of Pasquale, is a good innings by anyone's standards. In 1996, while working as an epidemiologist (someone who investigates disease), he discovered that mortality rates in the central, mountainous part of Sardinia were lower than elsewhere on the island. It made him think: might there be more people like his great-uncle there? His hunch was right. The rate of 100-year-olds was 30 per cent higher than in other areas and, surprisingly, there were nearly as many male centenarians as there were female. This was highly unusual; it's a long-established fact that globally women live longer than men (on average by five years as of 2021), a fact confirmed to be true by the World Health Organization (WHO) "everywhere in the world" in 2019.[1,2]

Not only were the centenarians in these villages in Sardinia living a long time, they were doing so in style. Fit, active, engaged, sharp and playful, these elderly people weren't dragged down, quietened or incapacitated by their age; on the contrary, they were living like those 20 years their junior and escaping the diseases normally associated with ageing, such as dementia, heart disease and certain types of cancer.

This astounding region of Sardinia became the first blue zone, a term that now signifies places around the world with the highest life expectancy, or with the highest proportion of people who reach the age of 100.

Genes vs lifestyle

At first, researchers thought the longevity of the inhabitants of the blue zones might be genetic, that these hardy, isolated, island folk might have a special gene, or version of a gene, that was protecting them, but when a 1996 study of Danish twins found that only 20 per cent of how long you live is determined by your genes, scientists started to explore the other 80 per cent: lifestyle factors.[3]

They looked at things like exercise, levels of stress, the structure of the community, what people did for work and, of course, nutrition. Had these people happened upon an ingredient with magical, life-extending qualities? Was the elixir of life to be found in their lunch?

Meanwhile, over in Japan, there was another curious place, a collection of islands that had long been known as the "land of immortals". In 1975, Dr Makoto Suzuki, a cardiologist and geriatrician, was instructed to start studying the islands of Okinawa, located at the southern end of the country, after the Ministry of Health, Labour and Welfare had validated birth certificates and other statistical data, confirming initial reports of the long lives and "outstanding health" of the citizens. He set up the Okinawa Centenarian Study, which is now the longest, continuously running study of centenarians in the world. There too, they took a close look at the habits of the people; how did they conduct their lives? What was important to them? What were the governing principles they adhered to, consciously or not? And, what was on their plates?

In 2005, with the help of a National Geographic explorer named Dan Buettner, the two longevity hotspots joined forces. Though they were more than 10,000km apart, with very different cultures, traditions and histories, they had a lot in common – and they weren't alone. Convinced there must be others around the world, Pes, Buettner et al. went on a mission to find them; first identifying Loma Linda, in California, then Nicoya in Costa Rica, and a few years later adding the Greek island of Ikaria to their list.

In these five diverse places, they witnessed the same phenomenon: healthy, happy 100-year-olds, uninhibited by disease and living their lives to the full. They were walking up hills, riding horses, playing guitars, cooking for their families and cracking jokes with friends. They weren't seeing out their final years sad, alone or ill.

We only need to compare this with the picture in the UK to see what a miracle it is. Unfortunately, while life expectancy in the UK has been increasing for the last 40 years, albeit more slowly in the last decade, healthy life expectancy – an estimate of the number of years someone spends in "good" or "very good" health as they perceive it – has not been increasing at the same rate, which means that while people are living longer, they are doing so in poor health.[4] This gap between health span and lifespan is significant. In 2018–20, a man in England could expect to live 79.4 years, but his average healthy life expectancy only stood at 63.1, meaning he'd spend the last 16.3 years of his life (*20 per cent of his life* in total) in poor health.

A woman in England could expect to live 83.1 years, but with a healthy life expectancy of only 63.8, she'd spend 19.3 years, or *23 per cent of her life*, in poor health, making the longevity gender gap not seem quite as desirable.[5] How does a whole two decades in bad health sound to you? It's a future nobody would choose. So where are we going wrong, why aren't we living like our blue zone cousins, and what can we do about it?

The nine pillars of blue zone health

Of course, there are those who win the genetic lottery. There's nothing the British press loves more than the story of 100-year-old Doris, celebrating her birthday with cigarette in hand, and confiding to the reporter that the secret to her long life is her daily glass of whiskey.

In fact, the oldest verified person to have ever lived was a

French woman called Jeanne Louise Calment, who claimed to have eaten nearly a kilogram of chocolate every week and only gave up smoking when she was 117. She lived to be 122.

People like Jeanne are the glorious exception whose stories we love to share, but you don't have to be a doctor to know that a diet plan of cigarettes and Dairy Milk won't serve you well. Besides, when the influence of lifestyle factors is so large (80 per cent), wouldn't you rather rely on them than on a small amount of genetic luck?

After years of studying the five blue zones, scientists concluded that the reasons behind the amazing longevity seen there are complex. There is a web of factors supporting their healthy ageing; one so intricate and interlinked that it is hard to distinguish one factor from another. Nevertheless, the team of researchers distilled nine common denominators that they believe are responsible.[6] They are:

1. **Eating mainly plants**: the bulk of the diet comes from nutritious vegetables, legumes, grains and nuts.

2. **Enjoying wine with friends and family**: in all the blue zones bar one, people drink small amounts of alcohol regularly, with food and in company.

3. **Not overeating**: the Okinawans, for example, practise stopping eating when they're 80 per cent full, which helps with maintaining a healthy weight.

4. **Moving naturally**, i.e. getting exercise without even trying, by, for example, walking to a friend's house.

5. **Having a sense of purpose**: in Japan they call this *ikigai*, or a "reason for being".

6. **Engaging in practices that defuse stress**, such as praying, napping or remembering loved ones.

7. **Having a sense of belonging**, which in these places manifests itself in faith-based communities.

8. **Putting loved ones first**, for example by looking after their ageing parents in their own home and committing to a life partner.

9. **Having the "right tribe"**, a supportive and committed group of friends who also have healthy habits that will rub off on them.

As you can see, three points pertain to nutrition. In researching this book, I asked all the experts I interviewed the same question: in the stew of longevity, how important an ingredient is diet? *Crucial, vital, key*, they said. Some went as far as stating with firm and vehement conviction that it is more powerful than any other factor.

They're not guessing; study after study suggests the enormous impact of diet on our health and therefore healthy ageing. In 2022, researchers from Norway set about quantifying it. They used existing meta-analyses (statistical combinations of results of multiple studies to draw conclusions) and data from the Global Burden of Disease study, a massive database that tracks causes of death, disease, injuries and risk factors in 204 countries around the world, the latest edition of which was published in 2020. They found that switching from a typical "Western" diet to an "optimal" one is associated with 13 extra years of life for men and 10 extra for women, if they began eating that way aged 20.[7] "Optimal" in this case meant a diet that "had substantially higher intake than a typical diet of whole grains, legumes, fish, fruits, vegetables, and included a handful of nuts, while reducing red and processed meats, sugar-sweetened beverages, and refined grains".

If – and this is likely – you are already past the age of 20, do not despair. Effects were still seen by implementing a diet switch later in life. By starting age 60, men could bag another nine years of life and women another eight. And it doesn't end there. Even making a change as late in life as 80 could add another 3.5 years to both men's and women's lives.

Amazing, right? To me it's thrilling to know that what you eat can have such a positive impact on your health. Firstly, the idea that something that's a source of fun and pleasure can also be good for you is an immediate win in life. Secondly, it's so exciting because food's remit stretches out far and wide: it is so much more than just ingredients on a plate or nutritional value listed on a packet; food is creativity, self-expression, history, community, family, the sharing of ideas and, of course, love.

The happiest diet

This book is called *The Happiest Diet in the World* for a reason. If good food brings health, then it also brings happiness, not just from the physiological effects, but also from the psychological wellbeing that eating, making and sharing great food produces in us.

Improving your diet and relationship with food can also

have huge ripple effects on other aspects of your life. For example, by embracing cooking, you can improve your self-confidence, which may benefit your work, strengthen your relationships and give you a boost in self-esteem.

Equally, just the methodical act of peeling and chopping vegetables or devotedly stirring a pan of risotto may punctuate your non-stop day with the requisite meditative pause you didn't realise you needed. In trendy modern-day speak this is called mindfulness.

Cooking is also good for connection, both new and old. Maybe you'll make a new acquaintance while chatting in a queue at the greengrocer's or maybe you'll fix a tiff with your partner by baking them a pie. Maybe the taste of super-rich mash will make you laugh at the memory of your auntie's insane butter-to-potato ratio or maybe the smell of parsley cooking in a tomato sauce will bring back fond memories of being at your nonna's house in Kent.

It is for these reasons that I believe that, of all the lifestyle factors that are thought to contribute to healthy longevity, diet is the best and most important place to start. It is probably also the easiest. While the idea of finding the "right tribe" or identifying your "purpose in life" may feel daunting or overly abstract, deciding what to put in your shopping basket is tangible and something you can do right now.

Just as food can make us happy and healthy, it can also make us sad and sick. Astoundingly, poor diet is now responsible for more deaths globally than tobacco, high blood pressure or any other health risk, according to a major study. Eating too few of the right things and too many of the wrong things accounts for one in five, or 11 million, deaths a year worldwide; which is 3 million more a year than smoking at

8 million.[8] This is not a happy state of affairs and begs the question: is what the people in the blue zones *don't* eat just as important as what they do?

The Happiest Diet in the World will explore all of this, distilling what we can learn about food and eating from these communities of super-agers who have cracked the code for long, healthy and happy lives. We'll go on a journey to their kitchens which, although in very different places and stocked with different ingredients, share the same broad food principles. We will look at what the various blue-zone diets have in common and, with the help of leading experts in nutrition and the latest science, understand exactly why they may be keeping them so well.

We will delve into fascinating topics pertinent to both our diet and theirs, including fasting, meat-eating, ultra-processed foods, sugar, wine-drinking, gut health, calorie-counting, fermented foods, the psychology of eating together and the incredible power of beans. We will also hear sage advice from those who have lived long and healthy lives. By the end of the book, I hope you will see your dinner in an entirely new way.

Why am I so interested in this? Firstly, I care very deeply that people eat well (it's the Italian in me); secondly, the moment I began looking into the diet of the blue zones for a piece in a British newspaper, I was thrilled to see something I recognised: the humble, simple, delicious cooking of my Italian grandparents – uncomplicated, good food that puts flavour first and is unswayed by the powerful pull of the modern food and diet industries.

No one in my grandparents' world ate to be "healthy"; they listened to the signals from their bodies about which foods made them feel good and which ones made them feel bad. Culinary wisdom was passed down through the generations to create nourishing dishes that they really enjoyed eating.

Unfortunately, because of our warped food environment in the UK, our instincts for what to eat have become obscured, our ancient wisdom regarding food forgotten and good flavour and good health disassociated. By examining the traditional diets of the blue zones, unpicking why they work and taking a critical look at the Western food environment, I believe we can reconnect with what we've lost.

In Part 1, we will look at the way we eat in the West: where we're at, how we got here and what it's doing to our health.

Part 2 explores the diets of the blue zones: what they eat and how this often runs counter to current dietary advice in the West – how was it, for example, that we got to be so scared of carbs? And so obsessed with protein? As for the idea that counting calories is good for your health…

Part 3, 'Old wisdom, new science', looks at just that: why the blue-zone diets work, and how modern research is validating the ancient instincts and practices that exist there.

Part 4 offers some practical advice on how you can eat a happy diet too – five simple principles which, if you can incorporate them into your life, will truly transform your sense of wellbeing.

Finally, at the end of the book, there are 48 recipes that prove that brilliant flavour and nutritious food are one and the same; truly nourishing for body and soul.

1

The way we eat in the West

Hayley's fridge

I opened my friend's fridge one day recently to find nothing but low-fat yoghurt, a "posh" ready-meal lasagne and some oat milk. I was surprised. Hayley is one of my most intelligent friends; the type of person who through genuine curiosity will educate herself on the topic of the day to such an extent that she could probably give a decent seminar on it, and yet the contents of her fridge were surprisingly misinformed. Hayley works out regularly, thinks about her diet and cares about looking after herself and had bought these items under the impression that she was making healthy choices. The yoghurt was low-fat and therefore apparently "good for your waistline"; the lasagne was from an upmarket shop, so was an innocuous time-saving convenience and "just like homemade"; and the oat milk, well, what health-conscious person would drink traditional dairy these days?

But the truth regarding the contents of Hayley's fridge is quite different and exemplifies what a minefield eating healthily has become in the UK and the West in general – America is even further embroiled in the confusion than we are.

What Hayley didn't know is that despite its wholesome, friendly packaging, her expensive ready-meal was nothing like the nourishing, homemade image it was trying to portray. Her fashionable oat milk (a dairy alternative so popular in the UK that Britons spent £146 million on it in 2020) might have invoked thoughts of a healthy bowl of porridge but was similar in nature to the ready-meal – a highly manipulated product containing added ingredients such as oil and gellan gum that your coffee could well do without.[9]

But it was her yoghurt that I was most intrigued by. Low-fat yoghurt is the ultimate symbol of our deep and long-standing food fog. It's not really yoghurt; it's actually imitation yoghurt, a persistent and powerful relic of an ideology that swept the Western world in the 1980s: eating fat will make you fat.

This easy-to-propagate message came from a study done in the US in the 1940s, which showed a correlation between high-fat diets and high cholesterol. Soon, American doctors were advising that those particularly at risk of heart disease might want to cut down or entirely eliminate dietary fat.[10] Once spawned, the concept that fat was a dietary enemy quickly grew legs, until people with no health risks were also starting to reduce their intake.

In 1977, dietary guidelines were published by the American Senate's Select Committee on Nutrition and Human Needs stating that too much fat in one's diet could lead not just to heart disease but also to stroke, cancer and, importantly, obesity. Fat was further damned in 1983, when researchers concluded that obesity was an independent risk factor for heart disease.[11]

Word quickly reached UK shores, and in 1983 we introduced our own official guidelines, which recommended the public reduce their overall dietary fat consumption to 30 per cent of their total energy intake and their saturated fat to 10 per cent. It didn't matter that the evidence behind the guidelines wasn't robust because the message was so clear, easy to communicate and seemingly logical: fat equals fat. Food companies had to adapt and the era of low-fat products began.

A clever and apparently simple solution was devised: just remove the fat. The problem is, when you remove the fat from say, yoghurt, a product where the fat content is elementary to our enjoyment of it, it tastes beyond awful. It's like trying to remove the meatiness from meat or the sugar from an apple; you're left with something vapid, bland and in the case of yoghurt texturally odd.

So they came up with another solution. To try to mimic the characteristic creamy mouthfeel of yoghurt, the manufacturers added thickeners and stabilisers, such as modified starch, which is starch extracted from grains or vegetables that has been treated to alter its properties. And to hide the strange flavour that resulted from this addition, manufacturers added sugar, sweeteners and flavourings. It was in this manipulation that the problem lay: to compensate for the reduction in fat, they had to ramp up the sugar and refined carbohydrate content – two things that we know when consumed excessively lead to negative health outcomes. In wanting to make a healthy choice, consumers had unwittingly swapped their everyday, healthy, full-fat plain yoghurt for something that more closely resembled a dessert.

Over time, all sorts of preposterous products emerged: low-fat cookies, low-fat ice cream, low-fat cheese and fat-free mayonnaise – foods that would have sounded nonsensical or impossible to our ancestors.

The late 20th-century war on fat had an impact on nearly everyone. I remember thinking it was weird that my nonna only ever had the "blue" full-fat milk in her house, whereas at home, we had the "green", semi-skimmed one. My mum was, for a time, also taken in by the influential low-fat doctrine, and even though I was a child I too had absorbed that semi-skimmed was good and that Nonna's choice was bad.

As well as fat from animal products, people avoided other fat-rich foods, including some that we now know to be particularly beneficial for us, such as nuts and olive oil. To make matters worse, because low-fat products appeared healthy or "guilt-free", people tended to eat them in greater quantities than they otherwise would have.

Scientists have since agreed that the demonisation of fat was unwise. In 2015, researchers in Boston concluded that there was no good evidence to support recommending a low-fat diet for weight loss and that people following them did not lose any more weight than those on a higher-fat diet such as the Mediterranean diet.[12] Yoghurt has been exonerated, with many studies showing that instead of making you fat, it may actually help you lose weight and improve your body composition, and the consumption of "good fats" (monounsaturated fat and polyunsaturated fat) found in foods such as nuts and olive oil has since been found to reduce the risk of heart disease.[13,14,15]

When it comes to milk, and in turn yoghurt, we now understand that stripping it of its fat is not without consequences. As Dr Tim Spector, a scientist who researches the gut microbiome, explains in his 2022 book, *Food for Life*, removing the fat from the milk removes other things too. "We stupidly believed we could just process the milk industrially to remove the fatty layer, and this would leave all the healthy stuff behind. The fat-soluble vitamins and nutrients get eliminated when you remove the saturated fat content, including vitamins A, D, E and K as well as healthy fatty acids like omega-3." Sorry, Nonna, you were right.

Tribal, confused and neurotic about food

And yet low-fat products live on, as evidenced by my friend's fridge. In fact, the question of what to eat has got all the more confusing due to the rise of social media: a Wild West in which erroneous and often dangerous ideas about nutrition are able to circulate like tireless spaniels charging around a field.

Enemy groups will state their food beliefs with absolute certainty and go to war with one another over them, resulting in a mêlée of conflicting messages. Those who subscribe to a carnivore diet will tell you that eating meat to the exclusion of all else will energise you and clear your brain fog; the gluten-fearers will assert that the protein that makes dough stretchy is universally damaging; and the raw food lovers will say that you should stop cooking your vegetables.

As a person wanting dietary advice, what are you supposed to believe? And why has the necessary act of eating become so intensely tribal?

"Food is up there with religion and politics in terms of our emotional and intellectual attachment to it," Gavin Wren, a food policy expert and content creator, tells me over a video-call one afternoon. Gavin spends a lot of time on Instagram, where he shares clear and engaging information about food with his 42,000 followers and also witnesses how ideological diets have become for some people. "Especially when you start looking at the specific dietary tribes on Twitter and Instagram. Whether that's vegan or keto or carnivore, people will fight for it in the same way they would fight for a religion or a political party and I guess that's because maybe on some level people do feel it's a life or death matter."

Gavin sees all sorts of unhelpful and sometimes deranged health "advice" on the platform, including, recently, a woman who was instructing people to stir their water with a glass rod before they drank it. This, she said, would "alkalise" the water which would "stop them getting cancer". Of course, the rod was purchasable from her kind self. "You get everything on Instagram from absolute woo nonsense like that, to people who are communicating genuine evidence- and science-backed information," says Gavin, "and everything in between."

To his annoyance, he finds that the evidence-based gang tends to be on the back foot. Just as with "eat fat, get fat", simple, snappy messages still have a shiny allure and are lapped up by people wanting to improve their health. "People want easy solutions like '*eat blueberries and you won't die this year*' or '*stir your water with a glass wand to prevent cancer*' but obviously we can't say those things, because they're not true."

As a society, all this conflicting dietary advice has left us in a bad place: confused, overwhelmed and neurotic about food. With each passing year we're getting fatter, sicker and shorter lived: after three decades of steady growth, our life expectancy began to plateau in 2011.[16]

Diet culture and me

The worse our situation has become, the more obsessed we've grown with weight loss. I see it among my friends, in newspaper stories about celebrities and on social media. In 21st-century Britain, diet culture is impossible to avoid. Luckily, when I was growing up, weight loss, or the avoidance of certain foods to achieve it, was never spoken about, so I remained blissfully unaware for a miraculous number of years – up until I was home for the summer after my first year of university and my local, straight-talking GP told me I'd put on weight. "I'm just wearing a baggy jumper," I replied. "I can see it in your face," she said.

Even then I didn't particularly care. The first year of uni, with its constant partying and morning-after greasy full English breakfasts complete with a side of chips, had been so much fun. But as time went on, I couldn't help but notice as various fads came and went. Some friends were obsessed with counting calories, others went on juice cleanses and one girl even told me, with stern conviction, that you shouldn't eat bananas or fruit in general because they'd make you fat. All this misguided tyranny would have been funny if it hadn't been so pervasive.

I remember very clearly when people started obsessing over gluten as the new root of all dietary evil. I watched a video in which an interviewer went round members of the public, first asking their thoughts on gluten – "it's bad" was the consensus, it makes you "bloated" and "fat" – and then if they could describe what it was. An awkward silence ensued. Each time a fad came along, I'd try and wheel back to what my grandparents had taught me about food – besides, I loved eating too much to ever cut out an entire food group. The anti-gluten trend helped clarify for me how nonsensical this concept was anyway. Of course, anyone diagnosed with coeliac disease should eliminate gluten from their diet, as should those who are genuinely gluten-intolerant. But the idea that gluten had somehow become universally problematic or "fattening" seemed illogical. Italy has the lowest rates of obesity in Europe and does not reject gluten.[17] Many members of my family eat pasta every day.

The obesity disaster

In the UK, on the other hand, the latest figures on obesity are cause for concern. As it stands, nearly two-thirds (63.8 per cent) of the adult population in England is overweight or living with obesity. Men are more likely than women to be overweight or obese (68.6 per cent of men compared to 59 per cent of women) and adults aged 45–74 are the most likely demographic, with nearly three-quarters of them in this category.

This national weight problem is a relatively recent phenomenon. Between 1993 and 2001, there was a marked increase in the proportion of adults living with weight problems in England and by 2019 the proportion of adults living with obesity had risen by 13.1 per cent. Average weight has gone up by 6kg and 5kg respectively for men and women since 1993. Sadly, it's a health condition that's also affecting children, with nearly a quarter (23.4 per cent) of all 10-11-year-olds now living with obesity.[18] The 2022 Broken Plate report, published by the charity the Food Foundation, predicts that more than 80 per cent of children born in 2022 will be overweight or obese by the time they're 65 and at least one in 20 of them will have died before they even get to that age.[19]

Obesity costs the nation nearly £100,000 billion a year (4 per cent of GDP) and is expected to grow by another 10 billion over the next 15 years as the population gets older.[20] Calling the situation a "disaster" in a speech to a Royal Society conference, Henry Dimbleby, who co-founded the healthy fast-food chain Leon before going on to become the government's food advisor for a time, warned that the NHS "will suck all the money out of the other public services" while "economic growth and tax revenue will stagnate". "We will end up both a sick and impoverished nation," he announced, gravely.

Diet-related diseases (such as type 2 diabetes, some cancers and cardiovascular disease) are now the leading cause of early death around the world. Our diet is killing us. So what exactly are we eating?

The Western paradox

The rise and rise of fake foods

The majority of our diet in the UK comes from packaged products that have undergone "ultra-processing". On average, we get 58 per cent of our calories from these products; among people from poorer backgrounds and children, the figure can be as high as 80 per cent.[21] At school, children can be eating lunches that are almost two-thirds (64 per cent) made from ultra-processed products.[22] We don't so much cook any more; we unpackage, we assemble and we warm up things made in factories.

There are levels of processing, of course, and not all of them are problematic – there is a wealth of difference between, say, tinned tomatoes and most pre-made pasta sauces. In 2009, a Brazilian scientist, Dr Carlos Monteiro, came up with a classification system called NOVA, which groups foods according to the "extent and purpose of industrial processing" – that is, how much it's been processed and why.[23] The groups are thus:

- Group One: unprocessed and minimally processed foods such as apples or cabbages – untampered-with things in their natural state, except for maybe being given a wash (which is why the word "minimally" is included).

- Group Two: processed culinary ingredients such as flour, butter and oil – things that aid cooking.

- Group Three: processed foods such as pickled, fermented, canned or cured goods like tinned tomatoes or sardines – things we've preserved to last longer.

- Group Four: ultra-processed foods (UPFs), which start to sound less like food and more like something you might find in a chemistry class. As Dr Monteiro explains, the processes to manufacture these items might have involved "the fractioning of whole foods into substances, chemical modifications of these substances, assembly of unmodified and modified food substances, frequent use of cosmetic additives and sophisticated packaging".

An easy way to identify foods in this category is by looking at the ingredient labels: if you find anything in this list, he says, that you would not find in a domestic kitchen, such as "high-fructose corn syrup, hydrogenated or interesterified [yes, that's actually a word] oils and hydrolysed proteins, or classes of additives designed to make the final product palatable or more appealing, such as flavours, flavour enhancers, colours, emulsifiers, emulsifying salts, sweeteners, thickeners, and anti-foaming, bulking, carbonating, foaming, gelling and glazing agents"... then you're in the realm of UPF. Do you use anti-foaming agents in your recipes at home?

In essence, UPF comprises ingredients that have been taken apart and reconstituted. Because these processes don't tend to result in products that taste very nice, chemicals have to be added to get us to eat them.

It is no wonder then that Fernanda Rauber, another Brazilian scientist, said: "Most UPF is not food. It's an industrially produced edible substance."

Unfortunately for us, UPF does a very good job at masquerading as real food. It can be anything from your "authentic" morning bagel, to your innocuous-looking "Greek-style" yoghurt, to the jar of curry paste you have in the fridge, the almond milk you're choosing because you think it's healthier or the protein bars you snack on after the gym. It's not just the neon-orange Doritos, multi-coloured cereal or the pack of muffins with a one-year shelf life; it's everything, everywhere, making it almost impossible to avoid. It's the routine staples you eat every day, it's the products that shout about their health benefits from attractive labels, it's your favourite takeaway sandwich and even your wholesome salad from your go-to lunchtime high-street chain.

These "edible substances" are generally high in calories but woefully low in and sometimes practically void of nutritional goodness. They are pseudo foods that you know on an instinctive level may give you a little dopamine rush for a matter of seconds while you're consuming them but won't make you feel good in the long term. There is mounting evidence to suggest that eating them, especially in the enormous quantities we do, is doing us harm; by fuelling obesity, depression, cancers, type 2 diabetes, cardiovascular disease and all-cause mortality.[24] Many public health experts have called the situation "an emergency". We will explore the impact that our ultra-processed diet is having on our bodies and minds in detail in Part 3, but we must first ask: why? Why are we eating so much of it? The answer is that it's so much cheaper than real food. The Food Foundation found that healthier foods are more than twice the price per calorie of less healthy foods and that a low-income family would have to spend 50 per cent of their income on groceries to eat the government's recommended diet – a simply unfeasible feat.[25]

On top of that, there is increasingly an access problem. One in four places that sell food on the high street are now fast-food outlets, where ultra-processed, calorie-dense, nutrient-poor food is available to people very quickly and at little cost.

"Our diet in the UK now, in 2023, is dire," says Professor Liz Williams, a senior lecturer in human nutrition at the University of Sheffield. "We have transitioned from a real food diet to one of convenience and we don't really know what's going into our food any more. Our food labels don't make sense to us." Even if we did understand the make-up of the convenience foods we eat, as the stats from the Food Foundation show, many people have no choice but to eat them. "There isn't equal opportunity to consume fruit and vegetables and at the same time we're bombarded with advertising to eat ultra-processed foods and go to McDonalds." There's this double-whammy effect of the cheapest, least nutritious food also being the one that's most aggressively marketed to us.

Overfed and undernourished

Maybe you'll recognise the counter-intuitive feeling I get when I eat a McDonalds burger or another type of ultra-processed product. The promise is big so I'm excited. From the pictures, the burger looks great; generous, juicy, meaty and filling with crisp, green lettuce for crunch, a slice of sweet, succulent tomato and a tangy sauce that will offset the richness of the meat and bring harmony to the dish. What you get is something shrivelled and pathetic-looking, with a single piece of wet, old lettuce, a salty, rubbery patty and an unpleasantly sugary sauce. As well as the disappointing taste, I'm left with a unique sensation of being both too full and still hungry. I can feel the slap of calories hit my body, like when you're paddling in the sea and are surprised by an unexpectedly large, violent wave. And yet, peculiarly, I feel like I haven't had enough. I'm lacking something. I've eaten, but the food didn't do the job I wanted it to. I leave feeling duped, disgruntled and thinking about what I can eat next.

This "I-need-more" feeling is a phenomenon we're experiencing on a mass level thanks to the warped food environment we now live in. We're at once overfed and undernourished, a sorry paradox affecting the Western world – the impacts of which are already observable in our young. Five-year-olds in Britain are now on average up to 7cm shorter than their peers in other comparably wealthy nations, the Non-Communicable Diseases Risk Factor Collaboration, a global network of health scientists, revealed in 2023. The average five-year-old boy in the UK is 112.5cm tall, compared to boys of the same age in Italy who are on average 117.3cm. The average girl is 111.7cm tall, while her Italian counterpart is 115.5cm.[26]

In 1985, British children ranked 69th out of 200 countries for average height but now, falling by 33 places, boys are 102nd, and girls, falling by 27 places, stand at 96th. Poor diet was highlighted by experts as one of the main reasons behind the notable fall in the league table.

How "obesity genes" interact with your environment

We're in a strange new world, where under-nourishing products not only exist, but have become completely normalised and actually promote weight gain.

A man who knows a lot about obesity is Cambridge University geneticist Dr Giles Yeo. Giles has spent the last 20 years of his career investigating obesity and the brain's role in modulating our food intake, and was part of the team that found the first obesity "genes". He has written two fascinating books on the subject: *Gene Eating: The Story of Human Appetite* and *Why Calories Don't Count: How We Got the Science of Weight Loss Wrong*.

A food lover, like me, Giles was quick to take up my offer of lunch to discuss the topic. After carefully researching the

Cambridge food scene online, I settled on a traditional Jordanian restaurant called Little Petra about 15 minutes from the centre of the city. It was full of diners despite it being a workday lunchtime, which was a sure sign the food was good.

"For the first time in the history of anything, we're now more likely to die of overnutrition than undernutrition," Giles begins, wide-eyed and serious as our starter arrives. "We're not getting enough of what we do need and we're getting too much of what we don't need." Calories have never been cheaper, says Giles. "In the UK you can get nearly 1,000 calories for 90p, but what are those calories?" Gesturing to the plate in front of us, beautifully arranged with hummus, stuffed vine leaves, fried halloumi, olives, cucumber, tomatoes, falafel, spicy peppers and pomegranate seeds, he says: "It's not meze."

While obesity is rising across the population, the fact remains that the pattern of weight gain is not homogeneous. So why do some people get fatter than others? For many years, the common perception was that some people were just greedier than others, that they had little willpower. It is not that straightforward, says Giles. It is not that some people have fantastic self-control and others do not; rather that our body weight is governed by a subtle interplay between our genes and our environment that we are not really aware of. The first influence over our differing appetites lies in our brains. There are three parts of the brain that are involved in our desire to eat: the hypothalamus, an almond-sized structure deep inside it, which tells us how hungry we are; the hindbrain, located in the lower back part, which senses how much fat we have stored and therefore tells us when we are full; and the hedonic region, which is the one responsible for reward; it is this that gives us a feeling of pleasure when we eat.

"The point at which we each decide to stop eating depends on the communication between these three areas," Giles says. For example, as your fullness goes up, the reward you get from eating tends to go down. But there are variations from person to person.

We now know that more than 1,000 genes influence these pathways and that gene mutations can affect our eating behaviour. For example, there is a gene called melanocortin 4 receptor (MC4R), which is responsible for sensing our fat stores. A mutation in the gene can cause us to perceive that we have less fat than we do, prompting us to eat more.

Such variations mean that some people feel hungrier, or take longer to feel full, or get more of a reward from food than others do.

In this sense, you could say that there are "obesity genes", but once again the reality is slightly more nuanced, says Giles. These genes indicate "genetic risk" rather than a guaranteed outcome, which means that, even if you have them, you might not end up with excess body weight. And why is that? Because of our environment.

Two people with the same genetic risk for weight gain could look very different depending on where they live, and it's even been observed in twins who are genetically identical. Giles gives me an example. "When I first moved to Cambridge in the early 90s, stores were not open on a Sunday so if I suddenly fancied a bowl of cereal on a Sunday night but had no cereal and no milk then, tough, I'd have to wait until Monday. Now, there's Uber Eats, there's Deliveroo, there are shops open. So my genes are exactly the same but my ability to get food is different." He can have his cereal when he wants it. This is what is known as an obesogenic environment; an environment which promotes weight gain and is not conducive to weight loss. And we have to remember that as humans, we're hard-wired to want high-calorie foods as a basic survival mechanism. When food like this is so readily accessible, it's hard to say no and before we know it, it's habitual and normal to consume it on a regular basis. We're living in a food environment we're not built for and can't adapt to – or, maybe we could, says Giles, if we were to wait a few millennia.

Are you enjoying that?

What can we do about this bleak situation? Until there is a major change to our food environment, which we should all push for, it would be nice to think we could at least do something on an individual level to improve our happiness and health. And the answer is, we can. The first step is to ask ourselves this question: what does it really mean to nourish ourselves?

While "edible food substances" cause a short-term spike of enjoyment, it's fleeting and cannot sustain our health or wellbeing. These products simply do not nourish us. Instead, they confuse our palates by trying to hijack the definition of "flavour", making real, nutritious, home-cooked food seem like the bland option.

I was always taught by my grandparents, indeed by my whole family, that delicious food and nourishing food are the same thing. What we will see in the blue zones is that this is the case and it makes everything so much easier. A fundamental factor in their good health is their enjoyment of their food.

They are traditional cooks who, because of their circumstances, haven't been influenced by "Big Food" or social media trends and "gurus". Instead, they have learnt to trust their own food instincts. They pay attention to the feedback from their bodies and their taste buds. They're not experts on nutrition – I don't think my nonna could have listed the micronutrients of her onion and herb frittata, but she could have told you if it made her feel good.

You can harness your food instincts, too

When you next sit down to eat a meal, ask yourself: does the food make you happy? Do you feel good after eating it? Are you really enjoying that?

In the blue zones, flavour is the ultimate guide behind food choices, along with freshness and availability, which luckily tend to align. I firmly believe that by getting back in touch with real flavour, which we can do through cooking, we can regain our instincts for what nourishes us and, despite our chaotic food environment, forge a path to good health. I don't think we have to search far into ourselves to know which foods make us feel well and which make us feel awful. Through all the noise, it is still there.

Furthermore, when "healthy" food is also tasty food you'll never tire of eating it. When you look at the diet of the blue zones, as we are about to do in detail, you'll see that it's not a quick-fix "plan" designed with a short-term goal in mind; it's a pattern to live by. With that in mind, it's vital to remember that if the food you eat does not taste good, you will not want to eat it. You can eat a dull diet for a while – a week, a month, maybe a year – but after that you will start to resent it and you won't have much fun in the process. I beg of you, do not waste your time with this nonsense. Let mealtimes always be an occasion of joy by realigning good health and good flavour.

To see how it's done, let's go on a culinary journey to places where food instincts still rule.

2

The diet of the blue zones

Carbs are not the enemy

When researchers started studying the healthy longevity of the Sardinian blue zone, their first theory was that it must be down to exercise. The men in this hilly, inland part of the island were mainly shepherds, which meant they did a lot of physical activity. Furthermore, the streets in these villages were particularly steep; people faced sharp uphill climbs to go pretty much anywhere – to the church, to the neighbour's house, to the man who sold cheese, to zia Gemma's for lunch. The result was that it wasn't just the men who were using their muscles but the women too. In fact, the scientists found that both sexes expended the same amount of energy per day, despite the men's very active work life.

The problem was, other communities around the world did a lot of physical activity and didn't enjoy the same healthy ageing benefits, so the team decided to interrogate something else: what were these people eating?

Perhaps these insular islanders were consuming something peculiar; something the mainland didn't have access to? A powerful foodstuff that either prevented disease or acted as a medicine for it? Today we might call such an ingredient a "superfood". Had they found the most super of all foods?

While there were a few unusual, local specialities in Sardinia's Nuoro region, the bulk of the community's diet wasn't coming from anything magical or rare; in fact, it was quite the opposite. One of their predominant sources of energy was a food that is distinctly unremarkable and universally consumed in one form or another: bread.[27]

It's no longer the main source of calories, but Sardinian sourdough bread is still an important part of their "remarkably frugal" diet, as is minestrone, a soup packed with seasonal vegetables, potatoes and beans that is normally eaten once or twice a week.

In 1938, a researcher named G. Peretti set out to investigate the eating habits of the region and found that more than 65 per cent of the total calories consumed by the population came from carbohydrates. As well as bread, they ate whole grains, pasta, potatoes and vegetables. Only 20 per cent of their diet came from fat, such as chestnuts, walnuts, olive oil and fresh dairy products from the many sheep and goats; and only 15 per cent from protein, most of which came from legumes, with meat, fish and poultry accounting for just 5 per cent.[28]

Though the Sardinian blue zone now has access to more foods than in those days, the emphasis on carbs remains. A 2020 survey found that the elders there report eating bread every single day.[29] The traditional diet is distinct from Italy's due to the high proportion of grains it contains; 47 per cent of the blue-zoners' calories come from them, compared to 38 per cent in mainland Italy. The diet still consists of very little animal protein – only 5 per cent compared to 10 per cent in the rest of Europe and 16 per cent in America.[30]

This may be hard to understand for a carb-fearing society such as our own. We've been conditioned to demonise carbohydrates, particularly bread, in a way that echoes our fat-shunning phase of the 1980s. And yet in my grandparents' home, it wasn't considered a proper meal unless there was bread on the table. We wouldn't just "carb", we would "double-carb", always eating pasta and bread at the same time. This wasn't considered indulgent; it was just our normal way of eating.

Why we turned against carbs

Low-carb diets, still ubiquitous today though often repackaged under terms like "keto", date back to the 1860s and to a retired British undertaker named William Banting.

Banting worried that he was carrying too much weight. At 5ft 5in, he weighed 91.6kg, or 14st 6lb, and had tried everything to get the extra weight off, such as vigorous exercise, bathing in spa water and "starvation", but nothing had worked. Eventually, he went to see a doctor who had recently heard a talk on diabetes and had begun researching the way different foods affect the body. He put Banting on a diet in which he had to cut out bread, butter, milk, sugar, beer and potatoes and eat mainly animal protein, fruit and vegetables.

It worked, and a delighted Banting wanted to share his revelatory experience with the world. In much the same way that the dieters of today evangelise on social media, he penned an open letter to the public, entitled "Letter on Corpulence", in which he detailed his new regime and its benefits.

His pamphlet was a runaway success, and his low-carb diet became so popular it generated a new verb; "to bant" remained in the *Oxford English Dictionary* right up until 1963.[31]

As diets go, "banting" enjoyed a pretty long run. It wasn't until the mid-20th century that a serious new contender was ushered in, with the popularisation of "low-fat" eating. However, diet trends, like all trends, are cyclical and by the 1970s low-carb was back with a bang and a new name: Atkins.

Dr Atkins' Diet Revolution, published in 1972, told its readers that they could lose weight while eating as much protein and fat as they liked, as long as they severely restricted their carbohydrate intake. Though not without its critics, the idea took hold and is still pervasive today. For my generation, the creed morphed into the catchy saying – "no carbs before Marbs" – which was coined by a reality TV star who believed it was her ticket to a "perfect" body for her Spanish holiday.

As we will see repeatedly throughout this book, villainising entire food groups is not a helpful thing to do. As much as people would like a single enemy to pin their dietary woes on, the fact is that eating, and its connection to our health, is far more nuanced than that. To get a clear picture of nutrition, we need to take a step back and focus on the overall design, rather than the individual brushstrokes.

Simple vs complex carbs

What people often forget is that many types of food are "carbs". There are simple carbs, which are effectively sugars that get digested very quickly, and there are complex carbs, such as vegetables, legumes, nuts, grains and fruit, that are digested more slowly and keep us full for longer. Complex carbs also come packaged with lots of other things that are good for us, including fibre, vitamins and minerals. Sweets and lentils are both carbs, but do very different things in the body.

In the blue zones, they regularly eat many complex carbs, and only sometimes eat simple ones.

Some complex carbs are more refined than others. Foods such as bread, rice and pasta contain less fibre than their whole-grain versions or, say, leafy greens or beans, and get digested a little faster (releasing glucose into our bloodstream more rapidly). Nevertheless, when combined in a meal with fibre and healthy fats, the rate at which we digest them is slowed and they're a perfectly healthy part of a diet.

The problem, in the modern Western diet, is that we eat a lot of refined carbs combined with simple ones (aka sugars) – think pretty much any supermarket-baked goods, pasta ready-meals or oven pizzas. A high consumption of these quick-to-digest, nutrient-poor products is bad for our health and is not the type of high-carb diet the blue-zoners enjoy.

There's bread and then there's bread

Take, for example, the industrially processed bread in our supermarkets; with its sugar and additives, it is very different from the traditionally made breads of the blue zones.

Sardinia is famous for its flatbread *pane carasau*, which is super-thin, and *pistoccu*, which is a slightly thicker version (and has the same etymology as "biscuit", French for twice cooked). Dry, crunchy, long-lasting and portable, these flatbreads were created to be the perfect snack for the country's hard-working shepherds. Both are made with whole-grain durum wheat flour which, unlike the refined flour in our typical bread, is a good source of protein and fibre.

The Sardinians also have a particular love of barley, which they use to make bread as well as other dishes. Barley contains significantly more dietary fibre than wheat and is particularly rich in a type of soluble fibre called beta-glucan, which makes you feel full and may therefore help you to lose weight.[32] A review of 44 studies looking at the effect of fibre on satiety found that beta-glucan is effective in enhancing satiety and that dietary fibre in general is associated with a lower body weight.[33] Diets that include barley have also been found to lower cholesterol, which can reduce the risk of cardiovascular disease.[34,35]

When they're not making flatbreads, Sardinians use the traditional sourdough method to make their loaves. They use a "starter", an active colony of wild yeast and bacteria cultivated by combining flour and water. When left to ferment, the mixture forms gases, which helps bread to rise. This is the original way of leavening bread and was used before the introduction of baker's yeast.

Sourdough bread has been shown to have less of an impact on blood sugar than industrially made bread; researchers believe this is due to the presence of lactic acid, which is thought to prevent or dampen spikes.[36,37]

Furthermore, if you struggle with gluten, sourdough could be an excellent choice. Anecdotally, people with gluten intolerances report that they can eat sourdough and the science backs them up. The fermentation process helps to break down gluten proteins, making it easier to digest.[38] This is why you don't feel bloated or sluggish after eating a proper Neapolitan pizza, which is traditionally made with slow-fermented dough.

N.B. Beware supermarket sourdough – much of it is sour*faux*. If you can, buy it from a trusted bakery instead.

Okinawa's high-carb success

Over in the Japanese blue zone – on the islands of Okinawa, south of the mainland – the Okinawa Centenarian Study made a similar discovery to the Sardinian researchers regarding carbohydrates. The population ate a diet that was 85 per cent carbohydrate, with a huge proportion of it (60 per cent before 1940) coming from a purple sweet potato that grew particularly well there. Known as *beni imo*, it set the island apart from the rest of the country, which relied on rice as its staple.[39,40]

Over time, this dominance of carbohydrates in the diet became known as the Okinawan Ratio: 10 parts carbohydrate to 1 part protein.[41]

With its high proportion of centenarians (68 for every 100,000 inhabitants) and 40 per cent higher chance of making it to 100 than the rest of the Japanese population, scientists couldn't help wondering: is a high-carb diet the key to longevity?[42]

A series of studies in animals has consistently shown this to be the case: a lower-protein, higher-carbohydrate diet extends the lifespan of a range of different species, and reduces signs of brain-ageing.[43,44]

Researchers even found that the Okinawan Ratio of 10:1, in particular, was the optimum ratio with regards to lifespan.[45]

So, remember, carbs can be many things. Choose them wisely.

Powerful plants

People in the blue zones mainly eat plants. In fact, when researchers studied data from Nicoya, Sardinia, Okinawa, Loma Linda and Ikaria from the last 80 years, they found that, as a collective, these communities got more than 90 per cent of their diet from whole plant foods.

A nice thing about mainly eating plants is that you get a lot of nutritional bang for your buck. They are nutrient-dense but not particularly energy-dense, meaning you can eat a lot of them; and eating a wide range of plants provides a variety of micronutrients, which is supportive of good health. The Sardinians have cracked this and manage it in a single, staple dish: minestrone, made with whatever vegetables are in season but commonly fennel, onion, carrot, celery, beans and potatoes.[46] Dishes like soups or stews are a great way of eating lots of different plants with varying nutrient profiles – like watching your favourite artist do a mash-up of their greatest hits.

One study compared the Sardinian diet with other diets in Europe and found that it contained far more vegetables, making up roughly 12 per cent of their total calorie intake, compared to 6 per cent, 2.5 per cent and 1.3 per cent for the average person in France, the rest of Italy and the Czech Republic, respectively. And this is particularly significant because vegetables have a much higher nutrient density than meat and grain. "Vegetables are less dense calories compared to grains, dairy, and meat, [so] a difference of 6–10 per cent in calorie intake from vegetables represents a much larger vegetable consumption than the number implies at first glance... Therefore, even when consuming the same amount of calories, vegetables are much more nutritious and provide a greater breadth of micronutrients such as antioxidants and vitamins, well known for beneficial properties promoting good health."[47]

A whole world of options

The good thing is, plants, as a category, is enormous. While in Sardinia the super-agers munch on tomatoes, aubergines and courgettes and make dishes such as *s'erbuzzu*, a brothy soup packed with herbs, wild greens, fregola (a pea-shaped, sun-dried, toasted pasta) and white beans, the centenarians of Okinawa enjoy bitter melon, daikon radish and seaweed, and make dishes such as *champuru* (meaning "to mix together"), a variety of stir-fried vegetables with tofu, eggs and soy sauce.

In the other blue zones, the story is the same. In Nicoya, a rural, mountainous and lush region of Costa Rica, the traditional diet centres around corn (often ground down to make tortillas), squash and black beans, as well as bananas, plantains and papaya. Potatoes are also an important part of their traditional diet and are eaten at least once or twice a week by many people.[48] Meat, fish and poultry make up only 5 per cent of the diet.[49] *Gallo pinto*, a simple dish of rice and black beans, sometimes topped with a fried egg and eaten with hot sauce, is a favourite.

Loma Linda in California, the most unlikely sounding blue zone, got its status thanks to a long-living religious group who reside there called the Seventh-Day Adventists. Having a healthy diet is a central tenet of their belief and, on average, they live 10 years longer than the average American.[50] They encourage a "well-balanced diet", which includes a wide range of plants – apples, peaches, avocados and mangos and lots of other fruits; a variety of vegetables such as broccoli, parsnips, leafy greens; many different legumes, including beans and lentils; and plenty of whole grains like quinoa and oats. Meat and fish make up only a small part of their diet and some in Loma Linda don't eat any at all, sticking to a vegetarian or vegan diet.

In fact, perhaps surprisingly, none of the people in the blue zones eat much fish. Researchers say that on average they eat up to three small servings a week and usually small fish such as sardines, anchovies and cod.[51] Fish is a complementary rather than central feature of the diet.

Finally, people living on the charming Greek island of Ikaria in the Aegean Sea love plants too. They have a particular penchant for *horta*, wild greens slowly cooked until wilted and tender, then dressed in olive oil and lemon. The Ikarians also make great use of an impressive array of herbs, such as mint, oregano, sage and hawthorn, which they regularly brew into tea, sometimes sweetened with a little bit of local honey.

A signature dish of the island is *soufico*, made from a variety of summer vegetables. Each vegetable is salted, drained and pan-fried in olive oil separately before being layered in a dish and cooked slowly together until beautifully soft, sweet and caramelised.

They're also big fans of chickpeas, walnuts and a special type of boiled coffee, similar to that drunk in Turkey, which they consume in great quantities. One study suggests that it might help improve blood flow.[52] Coffee may feel far removed from its original bean form when you sip your flat white in the morning, but it is just that – a bean.

Eat whatever plants you like

As you can see, there is no one magic ingredient; there is no superior vegetable that you must seek out over the others. These populations have different and distinct culinary traditions with a big variety of recipes that they hold dear and make frequently.

So the message is not *eat this plant* but *eat plants*. The power of their diets doesn't lie in the specifics and the idea of "superfoods" is normally just a marketing ploy. While it is true that some foods seem to be more conducive to health than others, none are so powerful that they work on their own. You could gorge yourself on polyphenol-rich blueberries, but it wouldn't compensate for an otherwise nutritionally weak diet of Pringles and Fanta Orange. It's not the *horta* of Ikaria or fennel of Sardinia that's keeping the populations healthy; it is their general pattern of eating which, at its core, is one based on plants.

I find this incredibly reassuring. Because it's a principle that's easy to apply to your own life, regardless of your location. You don't need to source Japanese purple sweet potatoes or Costa Rican *pejivalles* (small, orange fruits with a unique flavour that people describe as a mix of tomato soup, corn and sweet potatoes) to achieve good health – which is just as well because I've never seen them in Sainsbury's.

You don't need to buy expensive kale or try to source goji berries. You can buy frozen spinach and apples. You can buy whatever vegetables, fruits, grains, nuts and legumes are accessible and available to you. This is not an exclusive club with strict rules. Plants are a broad category; a vast, exciting world of different flavours and textures which, as well as being good for you, make life more interesting.

Meat as seasoning

It's hard to talk about plants without also talking about meat. In our Western minds, they're somehow seen as mutually exclusive, and are pitted against each other as if they're in some way comparable: *Do you eat meat or are you plant-based? Are you having the lamb burger or the one made of pea protein?*

Though eating a diet of plants may, in many ways, be the moral choice (and, for the record, I eat meat), the implication is that it's also the lesser one in terms of flavour. It's as if plants are the substitute, the mediocre back-up dancer instead of the star of the show. This has always struck me as slightly strange, since we derive such a breadth of food from plants and there is such a wide variety of meat that I wonder what we are comparing. It's apples and pears, or in this case apples and pork.

And why *are* plants seen as less tasty? Who decided that and when? And who decided that in an effort to try to make up for what we're missing, plants would need to masquerade as meat in all kinds of unappetising, ultra-processed creations? You can buy products such as "minced meat", containing water, pea protein, rapeseed oil, coconut oil, rice protein, flavouring, cocoa butter, dried yeast, stabiliser (methylcellulose), potato starch, apple extract, salt, potassium chloride, maize vinegar, concentrated lemon juice, emulsifier (sunflower lecithin), colour (beetroot red), maltodextrin and pomegranate extract), and something off-puttingly named "pieces" – pieces of what?

Why can't we just celebrate plants for what they are (delicious) and treat meat with the thoughtful reverence that, if you're going to eat it, it deserves? Plants are not a sad substitute and don't need to be manipulated into something resembling a chicken nugget for us to enjoy them.

In the traditional diets of the blue zones (and other long-living communities around the world, for there are others) plants aren't seen in this way; they're just food. Meat, which they historically had less access to because of its expense, is used sparingly, and generally reserved for special occasions.

In Ikaria, goat is slow-cooked into an unctuous stew, while in Okinawa, they braise pork belly with black sugar, soy sauce and awamori (a distilled liquor) until it's gelatinous and falling apart. These dishes are celebratory and the meat in them savoured and respected. My grandad had a love of slow-cooked lamb, which he'd stud with whole cloves of garlic and rosemary and roast on a very low temperature for hours. It was unbelievably tasty – all the more so because of the infrequency with which he'd make it.

In the blue zones they use meat, as my nonna did, as a seasoning – a way to flavour other food. In fact, this is one of the first things she taught me about cooking: using meat as a seasoning satisfies our craving for umami in the same way as actually eating the meat, and it's a brilliantly economical way to achieve big flavour.

I remember watching her put a single chicken thigh into a tomato sauce for pasta and letting it slowly cook away, infusing its meaty flavour. It added a distinct, identifiable depth to the sauce that otherwise wouldn't have been there. In turn, the piece of chicken would be transformed by the sauce; tasting incredible by the end and falling from the bone at the merest nudge of a fork. It sounds crazy that, as a family, we'd share a single piece of chicken, but that's what we did. After eating our pasta, we would have just a taste of the tomato-soaked meat before eating a big plate of salad and feeling perfectly satisfied.

In Sardinia's blue zone, the traditional minestrone, so abundant in greens, beans and potatoes, harnesses the deep flavour of meat by using pork stock.

On a recent visit to my nonna's village, one of my aunts, zia Camilla, instructed me to inspect a pot of bubbling sauce she was holding aloft in my direction as I walked into her kitchen. I had told her I wanted to know more about the way they had always eaten there, and the balance between plants and meat. Shrouded in tomato were random bits of pork: a small chunk of fennel sausage, a little piece of meat from a cheap cut and two bits of glistening tripe wrapped in string.

"It's an old recipe," she said, speaking so fast in Italian that it made my brain hurt trying to keep up. A recipe "delle nonne", or "of the grandmothers". Using meat in this way, she explained, makes for an exceptional sauce and nothing is wasted.

Once the flavour was just so, Camilla removed the meat from the sauce and deftly mixed it with some *cavati* that I'd helped my great-auntie, zia Pinetta, make earlier. *Cavati* are small, plump, indented pasta shapes, the perfect repositories for the slick sauce.

The sauce was as Camilla had described it: exceptional. There was a deep savouriness to it that you could not achieve with tomatoes alone. When we'd finished our pasta, she plopped a shimmering piece of tripe onto my plate. "It's not for everyone," she said, seeing my apprehensive expression.

The tricky question of meat and health

On average, across the five blue zones, people eat just 3.4kg of meat per person per year.

Compare that with standard consumption in the West, and it seems startlingly little. My friend's brother – and this is no exaggeration – once ate a 500g pack of minced beef in a single sitting; that's one big bolognese. Data from the UK government shows that this is not that unusual. On average, Britons eat 845g of meat per person per week. That's 44kg per person per year. To put this into perspective, the average chicken weighs around 2kg. This means that blue-zoners eat the equivalent of one and a half chickens per person per year, whereas Brits eat 22.

What to make of their light consumption – or our heavy intake? The subject of meat is a minefield for reasons that span ethics, environment and health. Camps in both extremes (devout carnivores and passionate vegans) will defend their way of life with a religious and sometimes angry fervour. There is always an expert somewhere who can back up a particular viewpoint.

Some commentators, like Dan Buettner himself, say there's no good reason to eat meat other than the fact that it tastes good. Others, such as Dr Mark Hyman, a physician who writes about nutrition and longevity, say it is the best way to meet our protein requirement, and some of our vitamin needs, and is important for a healthy diet.[53] What are we supposed to think as consumers? Does the blue-zone experience show that meat is harmful, or is their good health rather down to the fact that removing it quite simply leaves more room on the plate for beneficial plants?

I called Dr Oliver Shannon, a lecturer in nutrition and ageing at the Human Nutrition Research Centre at Newcastle University. "Meat," I asked. "Is it bad for our health?"

Firstly, he said, speaking in a slow and considered manner, it's helpful to introduce nuance. "There is more of a link between red meat and negative outcomes than there is with white meat." So, eating red meat sparingly is probably a sensible recommendation. Red meat has been linked to heart disease, diabetes, certain cancers and premature death.[54] It is classified by the World Health Organization as a Group 2A carcinogen, meaning it probably causes cancer – its links to bowel cancer, in particular, are well known.[55]

Secondly, dosage is important. We know that people who have a lower intake have lower health risks, so eating meat every now and then, as they do in the blue zones, is likely to be better for you. "You only really start to see negative health effects from meat when you're consuming it frequently," says Dr Shannon.

But what does frequently mean? As evidenced by my friend's 500g of mince with his spaghetti, we all have different ideas about the amount of meat we should eat. Within the scientific community there is not a consensus on a safe upper limit.

Dr Shannon's work studies the impact of nutrition on cognitive and cardiovascular ageing. He looks in particular at eating patterns such as the Mediterranean diet. The Med diet is built around vegetables, olive oil, fruits, herbs, nuts, beans and whole grains, and includes moderate amounts of dairy, poultry and eggs, as well as small amounts of seafood and red meat. It's a way of eating consistently linked to good health outcomes and very similar to the diets in all the blue zones.

Adherence to the Mediterranean diet can be measured by completing a questionnaire called the Mediterranean Diet Adherence Screener, known for short as MEDAS.[56] The questionnaire was originally developed for Predimed, a famous randomised controlled study set up in 2003 in Spain to test the efficacy of the Med diet. It's available for free online and it gives you immediate feedback. If you get a MEDAS score of 14/14, it means you eat a *perfect* Mediterranean diet. There are two questions about meat. You gain a point if you say you prefer white meat to red, and also if you eat less than one serving (100g of red meat, hamburgers or sausages) per day.

From this, and other data, it seems that eating no more than 70g of red meat per day is a good idea and this is what the Department of Health and Social Care advises. For context, one lamb chop is 70g and one small pork sausage is 50g.

If, for dinner, you eat steak on a Monday, lamb chops on a Wednesday and sausages on a Friday, you're pushing the limit – and that's not taking into account lunch. Another important point to note is that even eating 70g a day could be risky. A recent study run by Oxford University and funded by Cancer Research UK confirmed previous research suggesting that the more red and processed meat you eat, the higher your risk of getting bowel cancer. In this study, those who ate 76g of red and processed meat a day had an increased risk of developing bowel cancer, compared to those who ate about 21g a day.[57]

The easiest path forward might be to adopt a blue-zone attitude to meat, using it in tiny quantities to flavour other things, or having it every now and then as a special meal and really savouring it.

"From the evidence we have, I don't think consuming red meat once a week is going to be harmful," says Dr Shannon. "I think consuming it two, three or four times a week probably would be."

But if we cut back on meat, isn't it hard to get enough protein?

In any debate about the pros and cons of meat-eating, the word protein will come up.

My friends will often speak about needing to increase their protein intake. It's a notion that has spawned scores of products boasting of their high-protein content. Protein bars, protein powders, high-protein spaghetti made out of peas and even high-protein "Choco Crunch". Protein has become synonymous with good health. But why? Perhaps our protein obsession is in part due to our demonisation of both fat and carbohydrates – in a world where a lot of things we eat are "bad", surely one of them has to be "good"? It is also doubtless due to gym culture and the reputation protein has in that scene for helping people achieve "gains" – in other words, build muscle mass.

Protein is an essential macronutrient – our bodies contain around 10,000 different types of it. We use protein not just for building and repairing our skin, hair, nails and muscles, which are all made of it, but also to produce enzymes, which facilitate digestion; haemoglobin, which carries oxygen around our blood; and antibodies, which help us fight off infections, among many other functions.

It's undeniably important, but do we really need so much of it?

The Reference Nutrient Intake (RNI), put in place by the UK Department of Health in 1991, recommends that adults eat 0.75g of protein per kilogram of body weight. This means that if you weigh 60kg you need 45g of protein per day; if you weigh 80kg you need 60g. An average egg has 6–7g of protein, a tin of tuna has roughly 25g, half a tin of baked beans has 10g and a typical chicken breast (150g) has about 36g. So, if you weigh 60kg and eat a boiled egg for breakfast, a tuna salad for lunch and beans on toast for dinner, you've hit the RNI recommendation for the day.

In the UK, we exceed these recommendations. It's estimated that people aged between 19 and 64 eat around 76g of protein per day, with most of that intake coming from meat and meat products, particularly chicken. However, some people within the field of nutrition, such as TV doctor Michael Mosley, think that these guidelines are too low.[58,59]

He suggests we should be upping our protein intake to roughly 100g a day (15–20 per cent of a regular 2,000–2,500-calorie diet) in order to quell cravings and reduce the likelihood of overconsumption. He bases this on a theory called the "protein leverage hypothesis" put forward by Australian academics, Professor David Raubenheimer and Professor Steve Simpson, which argues that our ultra-processed Western diet is lacking in protein and therefore we overeat in an unconscious attempt to satisfy our protein hunger.[60,61]

When we think of protein we tend to think of meat, fish

and eggs, but there are of course many plant sources of protein, such as legumes, nuts, vegetables and whole grains. Instead of obsessing about the amount, would it not be wiser to be more mindful of the types of protein we eat? Certainly, diets such as the Okinawan one, which include mainly plant-based protein, are associated with lower mortality than diets that are centred around animal protein, particularly from red and processed meat.[62,63]

The Harvard School of Public Health concurs with these findings. They recommend considering what they call the "protein package", i.e. what other components are contained alongside the protein in any particular food – fats, fibre, sodium, and so on.[64] While lentils and a steak are both high in protein, the lentils are not a risk factor for bowel cancer and contain all sorts of nutrients that are good for us in other ways.

Let's step back for a moment and consider what exactly protein is. It is made up of various organic compounds called "amino acids". While some, known as "non-essential", can be made by the body, there are nine, known as "essential", that we can only get from our diet.

A common perception is that by reducing our meat intake, or going entirely vegetarian, we will be unable to meet our amino acid needs. But this is not true, as I found out when I went to meet Dr Federica Amati, a medical scientist and nutritionist, for lunch at a west London pub one soggy, grey Wednesday afternoon. "The truth is, we just don't need meat, especially if we eat fish, but even if we don't," Dr Amati said, as we both, coincidently, tucked into non-meat options. "You can get all the amino acids you need from plants; you just have to eat more of them."

Plant sources of protein used to be described as "incomplete" and animal sources "complete" under a belief that the former lacked some of the nine essential amino acids and the latter contained them all. This is not the case, says Dr Amati. "All plants contain all the essential amino acids, just in different proportions. Combining plants allows for the best amount of each to be absorbed."

While the amino acid distribution is less optimal in plant foods than animal foods, it would only really be significant if, for example, you ate a diet of only rice or only beans every single day.

In many cuisines around the world plant proteins are traditionally combined and taste great together: rice and beans, pasta and lentils, toast and peanut butter.

While you'll get a bigger hit of amino acids from a piece of meat than you would from a single plant-protein, combining them, which we do naturally, means you won't be deprived.

A note on changing needs as you age

There is some evidence to suggest that after the age of 65, meat, especially from good sources, might be beneficial. In fact, what we see in longevity hotspots, particularly Sardinia and Nicoya, is that the centenarians have started to eat more meat as they have got older – because their children and grandchildren do.

One study speculates: "Although meat products could be harmful before the age of 65, after this age the situation reverses, because meat may preserve the elderly from excessive loss of muscle mass, indirectly

> promoting longevity."[65] So interestingly, increasing your meat consumption later in life may be something to consider.

A sausage every now and then isn't going to kill you, but...

There is one thing we can say for sure: processed meat (things like bacon, ham, sausages, salami, hotdogs, corned beef and any meat or poultry that has been processed for preservation) is harmful for health if eaten regularly. The WHO lists processed meat as a Group 1 carcinogen, alongside tobacco smoking and asbestos. This does not mean these things are equally dangerous, just that the strength of evidence about their potential to cause cancer is the same. In other words, there is just as much evidence for processed meat causing cancer as there is for tobacco.

The WHO says that eating 50g of processed meat a day increases your risk of developing bowel cancer from 6 per cent to 7 per cent. This may not sound significant, but it is. Eating processed meat has also been linked to an increased risk of developing dementia, with one 2021 study finding that for every additional 25g of processed meat a person ate daily, their chances of developing Alzheimer's disease increased by 52 per cent.[66]

All that said, Dr Amati encourages calm. "Our bodies are pretty resilient. Many things harm us. If you look at the list of carcinogens for humans, you'll see that, bar two or three, they're all in our environment, so fixating on never eating a sausage again is the wrong use of your attention.

It's more about what you're doing most of the time with the majority of your food intake."

Invest in quality

If you enjoy meat, you don't have to give it up. It can be helpful for providing a big hit of protein and certain micronutrients, but the more of it you eat, the less helpful it becomes, and it can even tip over into being harmful. Think of it like a plunge into a freezing-cold pool. There are benefits when you stay in for a short time, but if you were to spend hours in there, you would be doing yourself no good at all.

The best approach is maybe to prioritise quality over quantity. What suits me is to eat meat only when I go out to a restaurant or about once a month at home. I save my money and always buy the highest-welfare meat I can afford because the idea that an animal has been raised in cruel conditions and endured a miserable existence upsets me.

When you use meat very frugally like my nonna with her single piece of chicken in a sauce, or like my grandad with his once-a-year leg of lamb, then you can afford to spend more on it. Investing in free-range meat from responsible farmers, of which we have many in Britain, will result in better-tasting meat than that which comes from intensively farmed animals, and some researchers think it is also better for your health.[67]

The lesson here is not to choose between vegetables or meat but instead to appreciate them both for their different functions in our diet and enjoy them accordingly.

Legumes for life

In 2013, Molochio, a small, quiet village dotted with olive trees in Calabria, a region in the south of Italy, hit the headlines. Among its 2,000 people were five, happy, healthy centenarians, which meant it had one of the highest proportions of centenarians in the world, four times that of Okinawa, Japan.[68] Scientists and journalists from around the world were intrigued and booked flights to Italy to go and investigate. It is also coincidentally the hometown of one of the world's leading longevity scientists, Valter Longo, whom we will meet later. Though it's not officially been recognised as a blue zone, many refer to it as such.

At the time, one of the eldest members of the community, 106-year-old Salvatore Caruso, told a reporter that the secret to his old age and health was "no drinking, no smoking and no women", but later added that his diet had been made up of local produce, particularly figs and beans.[69] Another resident, 103-year old Domenico Romeo, gave these thoughts on how to eat well: "*poco, ma tutto*" which means "a little bit, but of everything".

Today Molochio still piques people's interest and remains the subject of study for scientists trying to understand the key to healthy ageing. While they hypothesise and test, the village elders who live there now have some gut feelings about it.

Vincenza Celea turns 98 in July of this year, 2024. She has lived in Molochio her whole life, growing up in a family that she describes as "not rich, nor poor, but comfortable". Her father was a charcoal maker, and her mother, like many of the women in the village, an olive picker.

Her brother and sister emigrated when they were young, as my grandparents had done, but to New York instead of England. She stayed in Molochio, became an olive picker like her mother, got married and had her children. Now widowed, she lives with one of her daughters and her niece.

I ask her how well she feels in herself. Does she feel healthy, active, fit? "Very," she says assertively. "I'm in excellent health apart from some seasonal aches and pains." She looks it: soft skin, neatly styled, shiny, silver hair and carefully selected jewellery… this is not somebody who has disengaged from life. But more than her appearance, it's her manner that demonstrates her good health: she's quick, thoughtful and chatty.

When she was young, she'd help her mother pick olives for olive oil, she tells me, and she'd travel to the mountains with her father where they'd forage for food. She learnt to cook at the age of 10, preparing the simple dishes her mother taught her.

"Almost everything we ate came from the Molochio countryside," she says. "We weren't cultivators, but we bought all our food from local producers and cooked what was available and fresh. As a child, I ate only vegetables. I rarely ate meat, sweets, or fish. Meat was not a part of our family meals, even on holidays."

There was one constant: legumes. "My mother cooked them every single day," she says.

Dishes included pasta with chickpeas, pasta with lentils and *pasta e vajaneja*, which is Calabrian dialect for pasta with runner beans, a beloved recipe of the region that's still made today. It's not so much a pasta dish as a hearty stew with the addition of pasta. To make it you first prepare a sauce from garlic, olive oil, basil and cherry tomatoes and then you add the green beans, chunks of potato and sometimes courgette, before finally stirring in some cooked spaghetti.

Legumes were a lifelong staple. In the same way that some people eat bread every day, Vincenza, her family and her community eat legumes.

Let's pause for a second to examine the confusing semantics of legumes. All beans, including cannellini beans, butter beans, kidney beans and black beans, are legumes, but beans are also known as *pulses*, the dried edible seeds of a legume plant. This category is also home to lentils, chickpeas and dried peas (such as split peas). Meanwhile, fresh peas, fresh green beans, peanuts and soybeans – any leaf, stem or pod from the Fabaceae family of plants – are all legumes but not pulses. Legumes refer to the broad genre; pulses are a sub-genre and beans are a sub-genre within the sub-genre. Importantly, this whole category of bean- and pod-shaped foods features heavily in the diets of people who live for a really long time and they appear to be critical to their good health.

Certainly, a high consumption of legumes is seen throughout the five blue zones. Black beans are a mainstay of the diet in Nicoya; chickpeas are essential to Ikarian cooking; the Sardinians love lentils and fava beans (a variety of broad beans); in Okinawa they use soybeans; and in Loma Linda they're partial to pinto beans.

In my nonna's village in southern Italy, beans are eaten all the time. My relatives still chuckle about the time when as a very little girl, I was asked what I thought of the classic dish of *pasta e fagioli* (pasta and beans) I'd just been presented with. It's typical all over Campania, but each town, each person, has their own way of doing it. In the village they make it with white beans, onion, garlic and what in dialect they call *tagliarelle* (but others might know as *scialatielli*): roughly cut, irregular strips of fresh pasta. Chilli can be added, although it isn't for children, and Parmesan is a must. A generous helping of green-gold extra-virgin olive oil is drizzled on top at the end.

I took a big mouthful of my meal and chewed slowly, with a look of utmost concentration on my face, which amused the adults who were waiting, keen to hear my verdict. After a dramatic pause, I shouted: "Nice!" thrusting my plastic fork skywards upon my announcement like a tiny empress in my high-chair throne. Now, all these years later, the offer is not "*Pasta e fagioli, Giulia?*" but "*Pasta e fagioli, Giulia? Nice!*"

The multiple benefits of beans

Beans are nice, very nice, in fact, and not just for their taste. A 2004 study found that eating 20g (two tablespoons) of beans a day reduced a person's risk of dying by 8 per cent. The research, which followed 785 participants from Japan, Sweden, Greece and Australia over the age of 70 for seven years, all with their disparate food cultures, found that legumes were *the* "most important dietary predictor of survival in older people" regardless of their ethnicity.[70] No other food group was found to be "consistently significant" in predicting survival. The significance of legumes persisted even after controlling for age at enrolment, gender and smoking.

On the flipside, another study found that a diet void of beans may increase your risk of death.[71]

Away from death and dying and on to lighter matters

(literally), beans have also been found to be a useful tool for losing weight. In 2016, a review by the *American Journal of Clinical Nutrition* found that those who ate a daily serving (130g or just over half a tin of drained beans) lost more weight over a six-week period than those who didn't. Aside from the inclusion of beans, the participants made no other changes to their diet. The bean-eaters reported feeling fuller than the non-bean-eaters, which led them to eat less overall and therefore lose more weight.[72]

Other studies have shown the satiating effect of legumes. One experiment fed 43 young, healthy men either a high-protein legume meal, a high-protein meat meal or a low-protein legume meal. The high-protein legume meal was more filling than the low-protein one and the meat option. It kept them feeling fullest the longest and as a result they ate 12 per cent fewer calories at the next meal than the meat-eaters. Researchers concluded that it was the high-protein legume meal's extra fibre content that contributed to the feeling of satiety.[73] (Satiety refers to how full you feel in between meals, while satiation refers to how full you feel during a meal and acts as a cue to stop eating. Eating legumes leads to both.)

Another study of 8,229 adults found that bean-eaters had a significantly lower body weight than non-bean-eaters and a 22 per cent lower risk of obesity.[74]

And in 2020, a study which amusingly focused specifically on hummus (the delicious dip made from blended chickpeas, tahini, garlic, salt and olive oil) found that eating it made people less likely to snack on sweet treats later in the day. "Long-term trials assessing the effects of hummus snacking on health outcomes are warranted," the study concluded.[75] Fantastic.

So, what's going on here? Why are beans so darn filling?

You may have heard of Ozempic, the weight loss drug that's taken the world, or at least Hollywood, by storm, helping the rich and famous shed pounds effortlessly. The active ingredient in Ozempic is semaglutide, which works by mimicking "glucagon-like peptide-1" or GLP-1, a hormone produced in our bodies when we eat. This hormone sends signals to our brain to say that we're full, which is why Ozempic works – it simply suppresses appetite. However, it's not all roses. The long-term effects of Ozempic are not yet known but even in the short term, users have reported unfavourable side effects such as diarrhoea, constipation and even waking up in the morning with soiled sheets.[76] Glamorous.

Food, instead of drugs, may be a better option. Foods high in "fermentable fibre" (food for our gut bacteria), like beans, can trigger GLP-1, as well as another appetite-suppressing hormone, PYY. Beans have also been found to decrease your hunger the day after you eat them.[77] This is why when you eat beans you feel so full and are unlikely to overeat. If you want to lose weight, eat more legumes.

Legumes can influence your health in other ways, as well as how long you live and how much you weigh. There's evidence that eating them may help to lower your cholesterol and keep your blood sugar levels in check. Legumes are also a good source of protein that has none of the saturated fat of meat.[78,79] They're rich in a number of micronutrients (vitamins and minerals), including magnesium, folate, potassium, iron and zinc, which are essential for good health, and they are one of the only plant foods that contain the amino acid lysine, which is necessary for human health.[80] Like other foods we've encountered in the diets of the world's longevity hotspots, they possess the helpful quality of being nutrient-dense while also being low in calories. Which is the polar opposite of many manufactured foods so common in our lives today.

The beans that changed my life

If the impressive health effects of legumes have you searching your cupboards for a tin, I'm glad, but I think an even greater draw should be the joy of their taste and texture. Along with the *pasta e fagioli* of my nonna's village, there is a bean dish that I will never forget – and ironically it was served in a restaurant dedicated to meat.

In the fairytale hills of the Tuscan countryside lies a quiet village by the name of Panzano. This small place is home to a larger-than-life character, an eccentric butcher called Dario Cecchini, whom, if you are into watching documentaries about food, you may recognise from the Netflix series, *Chef's Table*. He has an extreme grey handlebar moustache which, if it weren't for his warm smile, might make him look like the baddie in a Disney movie.

With a couple of friends, we'd navigated the near nauseatingly winding roads of Chianti to reach his restaurant, a hill-top tribute to meat that attracts many tourists to the otherwise sleepy village. We took our seats and were quickly presented with plate after plate of beef; some of it grilled fast and some of it cooked slowly until meltingly soft. We gorged like medieval kings for what felt like hours until our bellies hurt and the room felt fuzzy.

It was a spectacle of meat-cooking, but as impressive and finely executed as it was, I came away from the experience concealing a terrible secret: my favourite thing about all of it had been a small side dish of beans. It seemed wrong after a carnivorous feast of such quality, but the beans were probably the best beans I'd ever eaten in my life. In fact, they changed my perspective on beans entirely.

Cooked until teeth-sinkingly soft but not mushy, cannellini beans had been artfully infused, but not overpowered, with the comforting flavours of garlic and sage. They were served bathed in olive oil and some of their cooking liquid, and they tasted outstanding – creamy, rounded and deep. I confessed my secret to my friend and to my surprise she told me she felt the same. "Those beans," she said, "were am*aaaz*ing." How great that something so remarkably delicious is good for your health as well!

Daily nuts

There is another nutrient-dense food that people in the blue zones eat all the time: nuts. Almonds are enjoyed in Ikaria and Sardinia, pistachios in Nicoya and nuts of every description are regularly consumed by the Adventists in California. Numerous studies suggest that eating any kind of nut is a habit that can benefit your health.

Botanically speaking, the definition of a nut is a little bit complicated. Some are dry, single-seed fruits that are encased in a hard outer shell that doesn't spring open when ripe. Examples of this are acorns, hazelnuts and chestnuts. Others are the seeds of a drupe, a fleshy fruit encasing a shell-protected seed. Examples of this are pecans, pistachios, pine nuts, almonds, Brazil nuts, walnuts, macadamia nuts and cashews.

Peanuts, as many people know, are different once more. They grow underground and are technically a legume.

None of this really matters. Culinarily speaking, nuts are oily, edible kernels that are incredibly versatile and nutritionally speaking they are *wonderful*, being rich in protein, healthy fats, fibre and micronutrients. They also contain compounds called polyphenols. This is a term that's popped up already. So, what exactly are they? Polyphenols are chemicals in plants that help to defend them against threats in nature and, interestingly, when we eat these plants the polyphenols in them help to defend us. They have an antioxidant effect in the body and, along with fibre, fuel the good bacteria in our gut microbiome. Polyphenols are thought to be instrumental in guarding against inflammation and there is even evidence to suggest they can protect us against diseases such as cancer, diabetes and other chronic illnesses.[81] Increasing your consumption of polyphenol-rich foods, like nuts, is undoubtedly good for your health.

A key longevity food

A 2013 study by Harvard that followed 120,000 people over 30 years found that those who ate a handful of nuts every day were 20 per cent less likely to die of cancer, heart disease, respiratory disease or any other cause during the course of the study than those who didn't eat nuts.[82] The participants were divided into six groups, ranging from those who never ate nuts to those who ate them seven or more times per week. Researchers found the more nuts the people ate, the lower their risk of premature death. Furthermore, they discovered that, contrary to popular belief, the nut-eaters were less likely to gain weight than the non-nut-eaters. As we learnt earlier, eating high-fat foods (which nuts are) doesn't necessarily equal weight gain.

Another, more recent study by Harvard found that regular walnut consumption is linked to greater longevity. Yet again, the researchers observed a dose-dependent relationship (i.e. the benefits increase as consumption increases). They found that eating five or more servings of walnuts per week may provide the greatest benefit; it was associated with a 14 per cent lower risk of dying from any cause, a 25 per cent lower risk of death from cardiovascular diseases and about 1.3 extra years of life, compared to people who didn't eat them.[83]

Yanping Li, a senior research scientist at Harvard T.H. Chan School of Public Health and lead investigator on the study said: "What we have learned from this study is that even a few handfuls of walnuts per week may help promote longevity, especially among those whose diet quality isn't great, to begin with. It's a practical tip that can be feasible for a number of people who are looking to improve their health."

I eat nuts every day because they have so much to offer in terms of taste and texture; whether it's walnuts on Greek yoghurt, roasted and salted pistachios or pecans as a snack, or literally any kind of nuts on a salad. They are essential for crunch and satiety.

And it doesn't matter what type of nut you eat. People are always trying to find a wonder nut, one that's better than all the others. It's part of our obsession with the idea of "superfoods" and fast fixes. However, health benefits are linked to all of them, so it's more important to eat what you like or a variety of them all.

But don't they make you fat?

The biggest barrier to people eating nuts is a belief that they're high in calories, and while it is true that they're relatively energy-dense, numerous randomised controlled trials have found that eating nuts, even in large quantities, does not cause weight gain. In fact, the opposite has been found. All calories are not equal, as we shall discover later. And nuts have been linked to increased satiety and therefore reduce overall food intake, which actually helps with weight loss. I'm glad that my fiendish peanut butter habit (the stuff that's just whizzed-up peanuts and salt, not a sugary, palm oil nut paste) is now condoned by science.[84]

Liquid gold

There are no superfoods, no superhero ingredients that can swoop in and save the day (your health) all on their own. But… scientists agree that there is something special about olive oil.

Olive oil, called "liquid gold" by Homer in the *Iliad*, has held an important place in world culture for thousands of years. What's thought to be the oldest olive tree in the world stands proudly on the Greek island of Crete, gnarly with the passing of what experts believe to be at least 2,000 years. Remarkably, it still bears fruit to this day. Could it be true that the fruit of this long-living tree extends its longevity to those that eat it?

Olive oil's usefulness has been understood and recognised for a long time. Greek mythology tells how it was Athena, the goddess of wisdom, who brought the fruitful tree to the world. She was in a contest with Poseidon, the god of the sea, to become the protector of a great new city: whichever deity could offer the citizens a more precious gift would win. In a huge and mighty gesture, Poseidon struck the earth with his trident, causing a salt water stream to appear in its place – impressive but not that useful as the water was undrinkable. Athena knelt gently and planted a tree, the olive tree, providing the people with shade, food, fuel and medicine. She won and the great city was named Athens. Since then, the olive tree has gone on to symbolise many things: success, vitality, friendship, peace and longevity.

Of its many associations, the foremost is health. The Greeks and the Romans certainly believed in the medicinal properties of olive oil. Hippocrates called it "the great healer" and wrote at length about the various ailments it could cure, from burns to cuts and infections. The golden liquid has had many uses throughout history. The Romans massaged it into their hair and skin as a conditioner; ancient Greek athletes rubbed it over their bodies to warm up their muscles pre-competition and provide them with an attractive glow; the living and the dead were anointed with it in ceremonies; excess supply that was no good for eating was used to fuel lamps; and in the 1950s, when my nonna arrived in the UK, it wasn't sold in the food section of shops but at the chemist as a treatment for ear issues and indigestion.

To this day, we still have a belief that olive oil is good for us and now science is starting to back up this ancient wisdom. Across all the blue zones it is the oil that is most commonly used, especially in Sardinia, Ikaria and Loma Linda.

What does "extra virgin" mean and why does it matter?

If you want to access the health benefits of olive oil you must buy "extra virgin". This is the unadulterated product – essentially olive juice – and denotes that it's been cold-pressed, which means it retains its nutrients and flavour. Anything that is not labelled "extra-virgin" has been treated with heat, which strips it of its health-promoting properties and wonderful taste.

"Extra virgin" also means the oil must be no more than 0.8 per cent acidity, a stipulation which ensures it hasn't oxidised, which would change the nature of the fatty acids and compromise the beneficial components of the oil; and that it has been subjected to rigorous taste tests by a panel of experts to check it's of the right quality. When it comes to buying olive oil, only the real deal will do.

I use extra-virgin in nearly all of my cooking. When I want to fry at a really high heat, which can evaporate some of the flavour compounds, or when the dish I'm making won't work with its distinct flavour, I opt for something else such as cold-pressed rapeseed oil or sesame oil.

You might baulk at the expense of extra-virgin olive oil. A litre should cost no less than £12 and if it does you should be suspicious. Olive oil is expensive because making it involves a long, laborious, manual process. I witnessed it first hand on a stay at a Tuscan farm, Fattoria La Vialla, one summer. First, you have to climb ladders and rake trees by hand with giant plastic combs; rather like detangling particularly thick and matted hair. You let the olives drop gently onto huge nets, which are later scooped up with great care so as to not bruise any of the delicate fruits, which would affect the flavour of the oil. Timing is of the essence. The olives must be washed and crushed within 12 to 24 hours of being harvested to retain their quality. As the olive paste is separated from the oil, both must be protected from oxygen and kept under 27 degrees Celsius throughout the whole process, including bottling. It's hard work but worth it. When considering the price, don't compare it to other oils like vegetable or sunflower – it is a very different product.

A complex flavour to rival wine

I adore quality olive oil and eat it every day. I put it on ripe, sliced tomatoes in summer with some crunchy sea salt and dip bread into the pool left on the plate at the end; I drizzle it on all of my pasta and vegetables and sometimes enjoy it on vanilla ice cream – trust me, it's a taste sensation.

I even had an olive oil cocktail recently at a restaurant in London, which blew me away.

For me, olive oil is a unique ingredient because there's so much complexity to it. There's the mouthfeel of the fat, which is nourishing and comforting, alongside the cough-inducing spice you get from a quality product. Then comes a tantalising tickle of bitter with this incredible freshness of grass and a subtle sweetness. Depending on where the oil is from and the season in which the olives were picked, there will be varying notes and sensations from artichoke to black pepper.

It sounds like I'm describing wine and that's because they are similar: single ingredients that offer huge breadths of flavour. Furthermore, thrillingly, scientists are now starting to discover that Athena was wise and Hippocrates was on to something: olive oil really is *astoundingly* good for you.

Midway between food and medicine

"It's a 'nutraceutical' product," explains Bandino Lo Franco, one of three brothers who owns Fattoria La Vialla. "That's to say it is midway between food and medicine." This might seem strange, considering it's a liquid fat (98 per cent fat) but Bandino recommends daily consumption, because the lipids, or fatty compounds, in it are of the healthiest kind: a monounsaturated fat called oleic acid makes up 73 per cent of olive oil, polyunsaturated fat, such as omega-6 and omega-3 fatty acids, make up 11 per cent, and the rest is saturated fat. Studies suggest that oleic acid, the main component of olive oil, is helpful in reducing inflammation.[85] In fact, the anti-inflammatory quality of olive oil has been found to be so potent that it works strikingly similarly to the drug ibuprofen.[86]

Though small, the rest of olive oil's make-up should not be disregarded, says Bandino. "The remaining part of its content, between 1 and 2 per cent, is composed of approximately 220 secondary metabolites of the plant and its fruits. They're minor but extremely significant components. Particularly worthy of mention are the high content of vitamins A and E (tocopherol) and the numerous families of polyphenols, among which are hydroxytyrosol and oleuropein."

As we know, polyphenols feed our good gut bacteria, helping them to grow, and have an antioxidant (protective) effect in the body.

Interestingly, polyphenols can communicate their presence via taste. "That spicy, tingly sensation on the tongue when you try olive oil isn't a defect," says Bandino. "Quite the contrary: it's a sign of quality, which is more evident in oils that have been pressed recently, and doesn't depend on acidity but on the presence of polyphenols, tocopherols and, to a lesser extent, terpenes. These precious elements are natural antioxidants; they protect the plant and fruit and, at the same time, are a panacea for our diet. As the months go by, the bitter and pungent notes progressively diminish."

As a general rule of thumb, the higher the polyphenol content, the more bitter and pungent the taste of the oil. The Italian chef Francesco Mazzei has this trick for identifying a decent olive oil: "If it makes you cough when you drink it, that means it's very good. If it just slips down like nothing, it's bad."

And what about longevity?

Never mind which component of olive oil does what – the overall effect is a good one, a very good one. A Harvard study published in the *Journal of the American College of Cardiology* in 2022 found that out of 92,000 people followed over 28 years, those who consumed the most olive oil (a tad more than half a tablespoon a day) were 19 per cent less likely to die from any cause compared to those who infrequently or never consumed olive oil.[87]

It reduced the risk of dying from neurodegenerative disorders such as Alzheimer's disease and Parkinson's disease by 29 per cent, from cardiovascular disease by 19 per cent and from cancer by 17 per cent. The study also found that swapping fat such as butter, mayonnaise and margarine for olive oil was associated with a lower risk of mortality.

"What was surprising were the benefits for diseases other than cardiovascular disease, which is already well documented," the author of the study, Marta Guasch-Ferré, told *The Times*. "And the fact that relatively large gains came with small increases in consumption."

At Fattoria La Vialla, Bandino's great-grandmother, Nonna Caterina, used to drink olive water, "*acqua mora*" (dark water), a very bitter by-product of oil-making, a couple of times a day during pressing season. She lived to be 98 and swore it was the reason for her vitality into old age. Since then, scientists have discovered that this waste product is overflowing with polyphenols; it contains 20 times the amount of olive oil itself. As Bandino puts it: "As often happens, our elders were right about things which modern times have relegated to the category of curiosities or superstitions." If you're interested, the farm now sells the olive water for customers to the public.

It can be difficult, as consumers these days, to know what to believe, with the hyping of particular foods (blueberries, quinoa, kale). However, the exceptional nature of extra-virgin olive oil is hard to deny, especially in comparison to other oils, so adding this ancient nutraceutical to your diet is a wise move.

What's the deal with dairy?

The scientists who researched the blue zones reported two points of interest about the inhabitants' approach to dairy. First, that goat's and sheep's milk is more common in their communities than cow's milk (they are particularly popular in the cuisines of Ikaria and Sardinia). And secondly, that this milk is often fermented into cheese or yoghurt.

What can we deduce from this? Should we all run out and switch our source of dairy?

"Dairy is always a bit of a controversial topic," says Dr Liz Williams, senior lecturer in human nutrition at the University of Sheffield. "Studies find it can protect against one cancer, but increase the risk of another, for example.

"It's obviously a really important source of calcium and for that reason I think most nutritionists you speak to will say it's really valuable." Just because the blue zones consume more sheep's and goat's milk doesn't mean that cow's milk is necessarily a bad thing, says Dr Williams. "They're just alternative sources of calcium."

While there are small nutritional differences between cow's, sheep's and goat's milk, what probably matters more is the quality of milk they produce. Animals that graze outside on a diverse mix of grass, flowers and herbs are going to produce a richer, more characterful-tasting milk. Just as we benefit from eating a wide range of plants, so too do animals.

In the case of the blue-zoners, not only do they consume high-quality dairy – often produced from milk from their own animals – much of the dairy they consume is fermented.

Fermented milk and probiotics

I don't tend to associate yoghurt with Italy. In fact, I never heard my nonna talk about it, or witnessed her, or any of my relatives in the village, eat it – it was as if it just did not exist in their food universe. That's because it didn't. Except in Sardinia, home to Italy's blue zone, which is the only region with a tradition for fermenting milk into a type of yoghurt known as *gioddu*.

As with many tales of food creation, the story goes that a shepherd accidentally left a bucket of fresh ewe's milk in the pen overnight. Having a quick taste before binning it the next day, he decided the milk was "*mizzurado*" (Sardinian for *migliorato*, which in Italian means "improved"), and so *gioddu* was born (the etymology of which is unclear). The fermented milk has a strong, tangy flavour (which is why it's also known as *latte ischidu*, literally "acidulous milk") and a creamy, slightly grainy texture.

When recently analysed in a lab, this ancient food was found to have a wealth of beneficial bacteria and yeasts similar to that found in kefir – another ancient, fermented milk, which originated in the Caucasus and is now having a moment in the UK – making it an important probiotic. Sardinians also enjoy a sort of fresh sour cheese called *casu ajedu*, rich in the bacteria lactobacilli.[88]

Probiotics are foods that contain live microorganisms (such as bacteria) that help to maintain or contribute to the good bacteria in your gut microbiome, thereby improving your overall health and wellbeing.[89] Prebiotics, on the other hand, typically foods high in fibre, act as food for your gut microbes and help them to grow. Pro = microbes, pre = food for microbes. Think, pro "in favour of" and pre "before". It could be that the Sardinian practice of yoghurt-making, unique in the country, gave its people an extra boost.

Raw milk vs pasteurised

Thanks to its many sheep and shepherds, Sardinia also has a long and proud tradition of traditional cheese-making using raw instead of pasteurised milk. Pasteurisation is a process whereby milk is heated to a high temperature for a set amount of time in order to kill off any pathogens such as *E. coli* and *Listeria*; however, these infections are unlikely to take hold if the animals are kept in clean conditions. Steve Hook, a farmer who sells raw milk direct to consumers in the UK, explains that the risk of pathogens is the same as it is for any food producer. "You have to recognise where those threats are to your food, mitigate them and validate your processes via testing, which is the same food safety measurement for any producer whether you're selling raw milk, burgers out of a burger van or a supermarket brand food."

The problem with pasteurisation is that it isn't selective – as well as eliminating potential bad bacteria, it kills off good bacteria, helpful probiotics that are good for our gut (and therefore overall) health. One study showed that children who drank raw milk were less likely to develop asthma than those who drank pasteurised milk and stated that the effect was partly explained by the higher levels of omega-3 fatty acids present in raw milk.[90] On an anecdotal basis, Steve says many of his customers report being able to digest raw milk with greater ease than processed milk, even people who thought they were lactose-intolerant.

Before pasteurisation, all cheese was made with raw milk, and advocates of the traditional method say it produces cheese that's not only healthier for you but also far superior in taste with more complex, interesting and rich flavours.

Gianni Mele runs a small family farm in the blue zone, passed down to him by his father, where his 300 sheep are milked by hand and their fresh, raw milk is used to make his traditional pecorino.

"With every taste you can smell the scents of the soil, the aromas of the herbs and flowers of the pasture and also the peculiarities of the sheep breed," he said.

"With pasteurisation there is a risk of obtaining a product with a flat, anonymous flavour, to which it is necessary to add various ferments and additives to give character. This does not happen with the use of raw milk, where everything takes place spontaneously, with completely natural processes that respect the starting raw material. Plus, raw milk is rich in living substances, which bring numerous benefits to the body."[91]

Raw milk is also an important part of the diet in Ikaria, a place known for its large numbers of domestic and wild goats that graze on a variety of plants. Raw goat's milk is drunk for breakfast or turned into yoghurt and cheese. It could be that this particular use of raw milk in the dairy production of both blue zones is important in explaining their health, though more research needs to be done.[92]

Deliberate sugar

The British excel at sugar. Our desserts – and this is a hill I am prepared to die on – are the best in the world. In a food culture that's widely denigrated for being bland or nondescript, especially when compared with those of our closest European neighbours, our top-notch puddings are something we should be immensely proud of. They are comforting, uncomplicated, bold in flavour and guaranteed to make you happy. They don't involve any of the faff or pretentiousness often seen in French desserts which can lead to a disappointing gap between expectation and reality; they're more satisfying than meeker Italian desserts (everyone loves a tiramisu but it's no sticky toffee pudding); and they're more substantial, more of an actual dish, than the bite-sized sweets of Turkish baklava or Japanese mochi.

Hot apple crumble and homemade custard; tender, crispy bread-and-butter pudding with vanilla ice cream; glorious trifle; and my nonna's favourite, a classic, old-school steamed sponge and custard. "A beautiful British dessert," she'd say. She agreed that while Italian cuisine was generally tastier, the British had really got it right with their desserts (a full English breakfast and angel cake also made the cut).

I think the reason I love these puddings so much is that they're actually very southern Italian in their ethos: the simple done well, a celebration of basic ingredients, making the little into something life-affirming. If you think about it, a crumble is conceptually akin to a plate of tomato pasta. The first is a fruit, plus flour, butter and sugar. The second is a fruit plus flour, water and olive oil. Both are greater than the sum of their parts. Both are like putting on warm pyjamas on a cold evening.

Before the French and Italians come after me, I'd like to give honourable mentions to some of their fine desserts too. Profiteroles were one of my first food loves – simple and yet stupendous. *Tarte au citron*, sharp with lemon and rounded with crumbly, buttery pastry, is a match made in pudding heaven; and Italian rum baba, a yeasted sponge soaked in syrup and rum, served with cream and sometimes Nutella, is beyond-words beautiful.

The point of this ode to puddings is to demonstrate that in a culture where sugar is increasingly being demonised, it is actually something to celebrate. It forms an important part of our lives and cultures, often acting as the centrepiece for our social rituals. Sugar is birthday cake with your friends, fresh lemonade in the park on a sunny afternoon, the sound of the ice cream van when you were a child, tea and biscuits with your gran and making jam tarts with your mum.

Sugar has gone astray

The problem with sugar in our modern food environment is that it's gone astray. It's no longer a treat; instead, it has crept its way into almost everything. Indeed, it has infiltrated our savoury foods so quietly and insidiously that we've barely noticed – we just think that's how things are supposed to taste.

For me the epitome of this is shop-bought pasta sauce.

In some parts of Italy, they put a little sugar into their tomato sauce and in other parts they don't. It's something that my nonna and grandad would often debate about. Nonna argued it balanced the acidity of the tomatoes, but Grandad was adamant that it was unnecessary and that even half a teaspoon would make the sauce too sweet. Grandad won the contest, and I grew up eating his version of my nonna's tomato sauce, without any sugar. I agree with him: tomatoes are sweet enough when you cook them right and sugar ruins the taste – I wouldn't think of adding it now, because in my brain it's just not necessary.

What's funny is that while my nonna and grandad used

to argue over half a teaspoon, the ready-made sauces we see on sale in the supermarkets, and that many people use all the time, can contain six times that amount. A 500g jar of Dolmio Bolognese Original Pasta Sauce, a popular brand that you can find everywhere, contains 26.8g or six and a half teaspoons of sugar. That's nearly two teaspoons *per portion*.

When I first tried one of these sauces, when living in a house with eight other girls at Leeds University, I thought it was extremely strange. What was this weird, tasteless gloop of sweetness? It tasted like an alien had tried to fashion "tomato" but had no real reference points to go from. Everyone else thought it tasted normal, nice even.

I'm not trying to suggest my palate is better than anybody else's – liking a basic tomato sauce doesn't make me a sophisticate. I simply want to highlight the unexpected places where sugar now appears in our diet and how, through continued exposure, our taste buds are getting tricked into thinking it's normal.

Our children eat more sugar than the adults of the blue zones

The Scientific Advisory Committee on Nutrition, which provides dietary advice to the government, recommends that "free sugars" (so called because they are not inside the cell walls of food, as in an apple, a peach or a glass of milk, but instead are either added by the manufacturer or the home cook; they also include the sugars naturally present in honey, syrup and unsweetened fruit juice) should account for no more than 5 per cent of our total daily calories, which equals about 30g or 7.5 teaspoons for adults. One level teaspoon is roughly 4g of sugar. Children aged 7–10 should have no more than 24g and those aged 4–6 should have no more than 19g.

The latest figures show that on average in the UK, we're eating twice this recommendation. Men consume 55.5g or 13 teaspoons a day, women 44g or 11 teaspoons a day, while the average UK toddler (21 months old) eats 25.6g or 6.5 teaspoons a day. By the time they reach the age of seven, that intake has increased to 57.4g or 14 teaspoons a day.[93]

Lisa Heggie from University College London, who conducted the 2022 research, said: "Much of children's daily sugar intake is hidden in packaged and ultra-processed foods, many of which are marketed as healthy. For example, a standard serving of breakfast cereal can contain up to 13 grams (just over three teaspoons) of free sugars, and some yoghurts contain as many as 15 grams (three and a half teaspoons)."

People in the blue zones eat just 28g or seven teaspoons of sugar a day, which means that even our children eat double the amount that the adults do there.[94]

Intentional vs unintentional sugar

This vast contrast in the consumption of sugar is one of the most striking differences between the blue-zoners' diet and what we typically eat in the UK today. They don't deny themselves sugar, shunning it as the latest in a long list of dietary evils: they eat it *deliberately*. They make a cake and enjoy it. It's a party, a celebration, a moment of fun and sharing. It's not an everyday event and that's what makes it so enjoyable. They know when they're eating sugar because it is in the correct foods. It is in desserts and sweet treats, not in bagels, yoghurt, cans of soup and tins of beans. In our culture the two have become disassociated.

Savoury food does not need to be as sweet as pudding. Imagine making a tomato sauce for four people and dumping in six and a half teaspoons of sugar. You'd never do it. Imagine adding sugar to your curry, your stew, your carrot soup and your chicken pie. The idea is unappealing. And yet nearly all our manufactured savoury foods contain sugar.

People of the blue zones don't have more self-control or self-discipline; they just don't have as many sugary foods readily available to them – it's as simple as that. If you had to bake a cake each time you wanted something sweet, would you do it? Would you whip up a chocolate chip cookie or go through the not-so-straightforward process of making and deep-frying doughnuts? Would you make yourself an individual pot of trifle or a caramel biscuit ice cream sundae on a random Tuesday night? I doubt it. We have enormous ease of access when it comes to sweet goods. If, on a whim, we want a white-chocolate-and-raspberry muffin, we can just go out and get one. In fact, we don't even have to go out. There are many services, especially in our big cities, that will bring dessert to us.

In the blue zones, which are for the most part rural places, putting food on the table requires a degree of effort. I was quizzing my great auntie recently on what types of things they'd cook in the outside oven when she and my nonna were young. She described bread, both loaves and flat (focaccia), vegetables like peppers, aubergines and artichokes and sometimes a type of homemade pizza without cheese.

"Did you ever make sweet things?" "No," she said, shaking her head disapprovingly. "At Easter sometimes but otherwise no, not at all." It wasn't because they didn't like that kind of thing; it's just that it seemed like a waste of time compared to making something more sustaining.

Why is high sugar consumption a problem for our health?

As the NHS website explains, eating too much sugar may lead to weight gain and increase your risk of related health problems, such as type 2 diabetes, heart disease and some cancers. When you eat, your blood sugar rises, which signals to your pancreas to release insulin, a hormone that helps clear your bloodstream of excess sugar and send it to your cells so that it can be used for energy. When you eat sugar every now and then, this process runs smoothly, for most people; but if you eat a lot of sugar all the time, you can overwhelm the system and your body can stop responding properly to insulin. This is known as insulin resistance, and over time it will cause your base blood sugar level to rise and potentially set you on a path towards type 2 diabetes and heart disease.

But even if you don't develop diabetes, having high amounts of sugar circulating in your blood for too long can be detrimental, explains Dr Federica Amati, whom we met earlier in this book. "If you're insulin-resistant, sugar can stay circulating in your blood for longer than is ideal. The problem with that is it's inflammatory. It stresses out your system." Inflammation is not bad when it happens at the right moment: it's our body's way of fighting viruses, bacteria or wounds. You can observe this in action, if you cut your finger and watch it swell up. This is acute inflammation and is a good thing, a helpful process of your immune system. The kind of inflammation you get from an excess of sugar, on the other hand, is *chronic* inflammation, which is altogether different.

"Inflammation is supposed to be a short-term response to tackle a specific issue but when it's sustained or systemic it's very draining in terms of resources," says Dr Amati. "It takes a lot of protein, a lot of amino acid, but also takes your immune system's focus away from what it should be doing, so if you get a virus, you're more likely to have worse outcomes because your immune system is too busy dealing with the chronic inflammation. Covid was a very good example of this."

Continuous glucose monitors

I recently became acquainted with my own blood sugar control when I took a personalised nutrition test for a story I was writing for *The Times*. It involved wearing a continuous glucose monitor for two weeks (a small device with a pinprick needle you attach to the side of your arm that reads your blood sugar every 15 minutes and sends that data to your phone so that you can watch your glucose levels go up and down in real time).

It was an enlightening experience and taught me things about my body I didn't expect. I am, what they call, a "bad glucose metaboliser", meaning that sugar will cause my blood sugar to spike higher than in other people. I observed one afternoon as it skyrocketed after I'd finished the last few sips of a sweet drink. The spike climbed and climbed and climbed on its steep and determined trajectory as I watched on my phone, held aloft in front of my face from a horizontal position on the sofa. I went for a walk, stomping furiously around the fields near my mum's home in Gloucestershire, to see if I could calm the volcano, and by the time I got home my blood sugar had returned to baseline in much the same way it had ascended, leaving an angry and intimidating mountain peak on the graph.

When your blood sugar spikes like this repeatedly, it can cause your blood sugar baseline to slowly but surely creep higher and higher – and then stay there.

Having the odd slice of cake will not immediately spiral you into insulin resistance or type 2 diabetes but having sugary food as a consistent part of your diet, repeatedly throughout the day (perhaps in foods that aren't even supposed to be sweet), and hence causing repeated and regular blood sugar spikes, is not good for your health. Let's be clear, though: this is about a general pattern over time, so please don't banish sugar from your life.

If you want sugar, eat real sugar, in real food, and enjoy it.

Artificial sweeteners

Reducing your sugar intake is a challenge if you have got used to eating a lot of it. However, the answer is not to switch to artificial sweeteners. Though artificial sweeteners contain no calories, they are not inert, and emerging research is finding they alter the gut microbiome in a negative way, adversely affecting our body's ability to process sugar, which in turn can lead to

> diabetes and weight gain.⁹⁵
>
> Moreover, aspartame, an artificial sweetener much, much sweeter than sugar which has been added to UPFs, no-sugar fizzy drinks such as Diet Coke and Pepsi Max, chewing gum and toothpaste since the 1980s, has now been declared a Group 2B carcinogen by the WHO. This means it "possibly causes cancer".

The curious role of wine

No one considers alcohol a health drink and yet research shows that people in the blue zones drink on average one to three small glasses of red wine every day with their meals.

It's a habit I'm well acquainted with. All my Italian family put wine on the table with lunch and encourage you to have a little bit "for good digestion". It's normally homemade and, let's say, won't be winning any awards any time soon. My nonna used to make it from grapes she grew in her conservatory in her little house in Kent and it tasted a lot more like vinegar than it did wine.

Back in the village where she's from, my great-uncle has a catchphrase: "Lil' bita wine?" He drinks half a small glass every day with his lunch. My great-aunt Filomena, who's 94 and very active and healthy, also regularly drinks red wine with a meal.

Alcohol is a Group 1 carcinogen, meaning it is a known cause of cancer, and the NHS states clearly that there is "no safe drinking level". Less than 14 units a week is "low risk" but not "safe". That's about six pints of beer or 10 small glasses of wine.

Except for the Adventists, the religious group in Loma Linda who abstain, all the blue-zoners drink some alcohol. The Ikarians in Greece enjoy their homemade tipple at get-togethers where they'll sing and dance merrily and the Sardinians sip on local polyphenol-rich Cannonau wine every day.

"Humans have been drinking wine for at least 6,000 years," says Dan Buettner, reflecting on the habit. "I'm aware of the World Health Organization's study that says there's no safe level of alcohol, but I can tell you that in these populations where people make it to 90 and 100 disease-free at the highest rates in the world, they enjoy their red wine – and in Okinawa their sake [Japanese rice wine]. We don't know exactly how wine interacts with food but there is one study that shows that drinking wine with a plant-based meal nearly quadruples the antioxidant absorption."

The mechanism by which red wine could be aiding human health is not yet known. It could be that when people drink it, they tend to be relaxing and socialising with friends (certainly, this is the case in the blue zones), and we know that genuine connections are very important for longevity.

In a study by the University of California, researchers found that out of 1,700 90-year-olds, those who drank two glasses of beer or wine per day were 18 per cent less likely to die prematurely than those who abstained. "I have no explanation for it," said lead investigator, Dr Claudia Kawas, presenting her findings at a conference. "But I do firmly believe that modest drinking improves longevity."[96,97]

Most studies have shown that it is red wine rather than other alcoholic drinks that is beneficial to human health and some believe that, like extra-virgin olive oil, it is its polyphenol content that is making the difference. There are 10 times the amount of polyphenols in red wine as there are in white, for example.[98] It is particularly high in a certain type, resveratrol, which comes from the skin of the grapes and gives it its colour.

Resveratrol is thought to increase the diversity of bacteria in our gut, providing many health benefits, such as reducing inflammation and improving our immunity. In fact, a team of researchers in the UK found that people who drank red wine had healthier guts than those who drank other types of alcohol. They also found an association between drinking red wine and a lower body mass index and lower levels of "bad" cholesterol.[99]

Another study from 2016 found that, after drinking red wine, patients with high blood pressure, or high blood sugar levels, experienced a boost in beneficial bacteria.[100] Other studies have shown that drinking moderate amounts of red wine may reduce heart disease.[101]

Some experts suggest that wine may increase the nutrient uptake of a meal: "congeners in wine combine with metallic ions, vitamins and fatty acids, facilitating their transport across the intestinal wall," writes one.[102] More research is needed.

Drinking moderate amounts of red wine is a recognised part of the Mediterranean diet, which, as we saw earlier, is generally considered to be one of the healthiest; in fact, in the scoring for the MEDAS questionnaire, you actually gain "points" for drinking about seven glasses of wine a week. "It's very different to the UK approach of minimising all alcohol intake," says Dr Oliver Shannon, whom we met earlier. "We know that the polyphenols are really good for cardiovascular health and also cerebral blood flow – improving cardiovascular health could have downstream effects on what's happening in the brain."

Dr Shannon also talks about a relationship between wine and food – the former's ability to influence the latter. "There is this really interesting synergy between some of the compounds of wine and some of the compounds of vegetables," he says. One that he's particularly interested in is dietary nitrates, found in things like green leafy vegetables and certain root vegetables, such as beetroot, which is broken down in the body to a gas called nitric oxide. Nitric oxide does a whole host of different things, but its key role is dilating the blood vessels. This not only lowers blood pressure but also improves their function, helping them to stay elastic as we age.

"We know that by having nitrate-rich foods, such as a bowl of salad, alongside a glass of wine, the amount of nitric oxide produced is greater. We think there are two reasons for this: firstly, the polyphenols seem to help convert nitrate to nitric oxide, and secondly, the polyphenols help nitric oxide last a bit longer in the body. So, by having a bit of wine with your salad, you see this nitric oxide boosting effect."

A "lil' bita wine" may indeed be helpful for our health when consumed with good food and good friends, but it goes without saying that drinking alcohol to excess is not good for us.

N.B. If you don't drink or don't like red wine but want a polyphenol-rich drink, then stick the kettle on. Tea, of many different types, is also full of the beneficial plant chemicals – the Ikarians drink homemade herbal tea all day long, but even a good, old cup of English Breakfast will do.

3

Old wisdom, new science

When it comes to eating well, I'm a big believer in both individual instinct and the collective power of culinary wisdom. I think that the things we intuit about nutrition tend to hold true and that old recipes, traditions and techniques that are passed down through the generations are usually pleasing not only in terms of taste but also in terms of health.

In this part of the book, we're going to explore the amazing science that has come out in recent years that explains the diet of the blue zones, and underlines the good sense of all sorts of ancient practices and instincts that have sustained populations for centuries but that we are now increasingly in danger of forgetting.

Let's jump in.

Fasting and longevity

"There is nothing as effective as nutrition and fasting for living longer," says Professor Valter Longo over the phone from Los Angeles. "It's hard to think of anything that even comes close. In fact, if you took 100 of the world's leading scientists in longevity and asked, *what could I do now to live longer*, almost everyone would say the number one thing is nutrition."

Valter Longo is one of those leading scientists in longevity. He's a professor of gerontology and biological sciences and director of both the Longevity Institute at the University of Southern California and the Longevity and Cancer Program at the IFOM Institute of Molecular Oncology in Milan, Italy. But he is also, as I mentioned above, originally from the little Calabrian village of Molochio, one of the world's longevity hotspots.

He'd already been researching how nutrition affects ageing when he realised a place that might hold the answers was right in front of his nose.

"I never thought to study Molochio because it's my home, but when I realised there were one, two, three, four, five centenarians all living there at once, in that tiny place, I thought I had to take a look." Since then, he's been investigating the reasons behind the remarkable longevity of the village.

He'd become interested in ageing a long time ago; in fact, the life event that sparked his fascination with the topic happened when he was a boy. "I was in the room when my grandfather died," he tells me. He was five years old at the time. "You're not normally in the room for that kind of thing but I happened to be and it's something that really stuck with me. My grandfather was there and then he was gone. It clarified to me that there was nothing more important – I knew I had to study ageing. As I grew up the drive was very strong."

In his village, as he knew, people ate in a simple way, making particular use of the local produce that grew in abundance. In general, their diet consisted of vegetables, pasta, olive oil, legumes, nuts, such as walnuts, which they picked off the trees, fruit, potatoes, a tiny bit of meat when they could afford it and a little dairy mainly from goats.

Their healthy diet wasn't on purpose but just a happy accident of their surroundings. "None of the places I've visited, Okinawa etc, have ever been trying to achieve longevity – with the exception of Loma Linda, where having a healthy diet is important in their religion – they were just poor and had the same food over and over; it turns out that food was the right food."

Calorie restriction and lifespan

But there was another factor that Professor Longo observed in Molochio that he believes is crucial to their long lives and good health: not just what they eat, but the quantity.

It's an intriguing phenomenon that we've witnessed in animals for many years. For decades, research has shown that calorie restriction dramatically boosts the lifespan of a wide range of different species, from monkeys and rats, to flies, worms, dogs, fish and yeast, as long as their nutritional needs are still met. No other anti-ageing intervention has come anywhere close in terms of effect and consistency of results.

This curious fact was first discovered in 1935 by a scientist named Clive McCay, who was startled to find that severely restricting rats' diets caused them to live 33 per cent longer than ever known to be possible. Since then, similar experiments have been conducted with other animals and have shown incredible life-extending results of between 50 and 300 per cent.[103] Rhesus monkeys that had their calories cut by 30 per cent not only lived longer than a control group, who could eat with abandon, but were less likely to develop age-related disease such as diabetes, cancer, heart conditions and cognitive decline.[104] A captivating photo from the study shows two monkeys side by side; on the left, one from the restricted calorie group, and on the right, one from the control category. The monkey on the right holds himself upright and looks strong, lean, muscular and alert, but the other, who could eat to his heart's content, looks like a frail, little, old man: hunched over with tired eyes and drooping, saggy skin on his chest and a visibly older face, wrinkled like a human being.

When Professor Longo began to investigate longevity in Molochio, he realised the villagers had also undergone a form of calorie restriction, though not intentionally. "Many of the centenarians there had been through the war where they had little to no food and other times besides the war where they struggled to have enough to eat. Then there were decades where they'd eat the same thing over and over – it was normally *pasta e vajaneja*, pasta with green beans. And then eventually when they got to 80 or 90, they'd move in with their children, where they began eating more, which was consistent with epidemiological data but also our mice studies that [showed that] restricted diets seem to be very important for the majority of adult life but then as one gets older a very restricted diet is no longer beneficial. So, from that we propose that there are multiple phases of eating in our lives – one in particular where you should be restricted, followed by one where you should not be as restricted and eat more animal products."

Giovanna Trimarchi, 93, is testament to this particular diet and these peculiar phases of eating. "I didn't eat normally for many years during the war," she recalls, speaking to me from her home in Molochio via video-call. "There was no bread or meat; for three years all we had to eat were oranges and lupini beans. I remember being very hungry and eating a lot of oranges." When the war ended and normal food production could resume, she consumed the fruits of the land – mainly beans, potatoes and vegetables – but because of her job as an olive picker she would often go without lunch. Now, many years later, she eats more meat than she used to, influenced by her children's habits; but even now she never overeats. "I think it's important to eat the right portion. I think that you need to eat less to live longer."

Vincenza Celea remembers the same thing: "There were times during the war when we had only one meal for several days, or even days without food."

Another resident, Angelo Matarozzo, 95, still purposefully doesn't overindulge: "Always leave the table with a bit of hunger," he says.

The other blue zones have similar practices. In Ikaria, Dr Christina Chrysohoou, a cardiologist who studied the diet and lifestyle habits of the islanders in 2009, concluded that while their plant-rich diet was good for them, she believed that the most important thing was that "they consume small quantities of food in each serving; in that way they take in much lower calories than we do".[105]

Okinawans have a saying: "*hara hachi bu*", which reminds them to stop eating when their stomachs are 80 per cent full. In Nicoya, they do the bulk of their eating early in the day and only have a very light evening meal or nothing at all. Research found that Nicoyans eat fewer calories than people in the rest of Costa Rica.[106]

It sounds counter-intuitive that eating less food, the substance we need to survive, leads to longer lives, so how exactly does it work?

A system reboot

"The number one way to protect against disease is by tackling the ageing process," says Professor Longo. "If you lower your biological age by five years you will cut the risk of Alzheimer's in half, for example. Ageing is really in charge of lots of the diseases; not all of them, obviously, but lots of them." So if you slow or reverse ageing, you can protect yourself against disease. It all sounds very sci-fi, but it's not.

Professor Longo says an easy way to understand how nutrition affects ageing is to examine a simple organism like yeast. There are three modalities, he explains. If yeast has a lot of food it stays in "phase one" and lives three or four days. If its food source decreases, it goes into something called the "stationary" phase and lives up to two weeks – a fivefold increase in lifespan. Then, if it's really starving, it enters the next phase and can live for years. "There's a 100-fold difference in the lifespan of yeast based on its nutritional condition. Nutrition determines what phase one is in – a high-growth state or a maintenance mode."

Then Professor Longo discovered that it wasn't just the fasting that was important but also the "re-feeding". "Essentially, when you fast an organism, be it yeast, a rat or a human being, it'll shrink and in that shrinking process it gets rid of a lot of junk at a cellular and intracellular level," he explains. "Eventually, stem cells start proliferating or normal cells are reprogrammed to become like stem cells."

When you re-feed, i.e. you eat again, you see an "expansion" in all the systems. "We've shown this in the gut, in the liver, the muscles, the blood system, the brain – it's a multisystem effect. In this process, you have a rejuvenation of all the systems." Like a big clean-up and reboot of the system?, I ask. "More like a clean-up and replacement. You clean it up, you break it down and you replace it," he says. It's like doing a spring clean of your wardrobe where you bin some old jumpers and buy new ones.

His work on mice has shown that fasting has a tremendous effect, extending their lives, lowering their incidence of cancer and delaying cognitive decline.

Mimicking fasting

You may not like the sound of fasting – not many people do – and being aware of that, Professor Longo came up with a clever solution: to mimic the process while still being able to eat. In 2008, he and his team discovered that water-only fasting makes mice much more resistant to chemotherapy and cancer cells more sensitive to it. Human patients, however, didn't like the idea of having only water, so, thanks to funding from the Italian government, he devised a diet that produces a response that mimics fasting in the body. "It started off for cancer patients, but then we tested it on many different diseases and people without a disease with positive results."

It's a low-protein, low-sugar, low-calorie, high-fat, vegan diet that you follow for four or five days at a time. "It's a lot of vegetables, nuts, olive oil, herbal tea." A study of healthy adults who followed the fast-mimicking diet for a five-day stint for three consecutive months found that it reduced fasting blood sugar, body weight, body fat, blood pressure and C-reactive protein (a measure of inflammation in the body). In another small human trial, published in February 2024,

Professor Longo and his team found that three rounds of the fast-mimicking diet can reverse biological age by up to 2.5 years.[107]

Professor Longo is now in the process of testing the diet again on 500 volunteers from Molochio. One group will eat a longevity diet (like the village elders have always done, with a focus on plant-based foods and some fish) and do the fast-mimicking diet every three months; another group will eat what they please and do the fast-mimicking diet every three months; and the other group will act as the control.

"Even if you have a terrible diet, if you're exposed to five days of a low-calorie, vegan diet, it's an opportunity for your brain to associate it with wellbeing – training the brain to say, *I want to be in that state*." It's like when you go for a run, he says. Things happen in your brain that make you feel good, so it's not so much your logical mind deciding to put your trainers on again but your unconscious deciding you want more of that wellbeing state.

"The clinical trials are suggesting that if someone's 55 you're not going to make them 25 again but you are going to make them much more functional and in most patients we see them return to a much healthier state than when they started."

Live to 100? Why not?

Professor Longo remembers his grandfather often, especially in comparison to one of his peers in the village, Salvatore Caruso, who lived to be 110, making him, at one point, the oldest man in Europe. "They were born at roughly the same time but by the time Salvatore died, my grandfather had already been dead for 40 years." He died from a hernia that could have been treated had he gone to the doctor.

People need to start realising that living to 100, still healthy, is an achievable goal, says Professor Longo. "Soon enough, we'll have two populations in the world. Half a billion who do all the right things, follow all the real experts and will probably on average live to 100 and others who go in the other direction and just don't care. These people will probably have a shorter lifespan than we have now. We're already starting to see lifespan decrease in the US."

Even Molochio, with its decades of tradition of eating well, has started to see changes in the diet and in the health of its population. "The prevalence of overweight people in Calabria now is so bad it surpasses America. We're starting to see children with type 2 diabetes."

I'm shocked, I say. I thought the love of the traditional cuisine would have prevailed. "That works until McDonalds moves in. And the medical system doesn't really mind because that's a lot of clients. Food is the number one way to get cancer, cardiovascular disease, diabetes, Alzheimer's. If you're diabetic, you almost double your chances of getting Alzheimer's. That's just the perfect system for a lot of companies to make a lot of money so nobody wants to change it. Things are getting worse and worse and worse – both the type of food and the amount of it. We're seeing it everywhere – India, South America, Central America, the Middle East. Bad food is like cancer, it spreads rapidly."

What, if anything, can we do about this? Eat like the elderly *molochiesi*, says Professor Longo, and practise periodic fasting. "Maybe in the future we'll come up with a miracle medical intervention but for now nutrition is number one, exercise is number two."

Feeding windows

If the idea of a five-day-long fast doesn't appeal to you, there is some evidence to suggest that cutting down your "feeding window" (horrible term) and hence extending your overnight fast might have merit. Previously, scientists were unable to distinguish whether benefits came from calorie restriction alone or if the act of not eating for an extended period was the key.

A study published in *Science* in 2022 found a way to separate the two.[108] Mice were split into six groups: the control group had plentiful food available 24 hours a day, while the other five groups had their calories restricted by 30 per cent. Two of these groups were fed at night time (peak activity time for these nocturnal creatures); one had a 12-hour feeding window, the other just a two-hour feeding window. These two groups lived longer than all the other groups and 35 per cent longer than the control.

The researchers concluded that "caloric restriction extended lifespan as expected, but it worked best when feeding was restricted so that the animals fasted for at least 12 hours and when the period in which the animals ate corresponded to the active phase of their circadian cycle."

The implication is that it's not just eating less that's important; it's fasting and doing so at the right time of day. Because humans are not nocturnal like mice, the right time for us to fast is overnight, as we do naturally, and there is evidence to suggest that extending this fasting period would be beneficial. A 2023 study by Dr Sarah Berry at King's College London found that eating in a 10-hour window (and fasting for 14 hours) resulted in higher energy, better mood and lower hunger levels. In practice, this would look like doing all your eating for the day between 9am and 7pm.[109]

The elderly folk of the blue zones all feel that not over-indulging themselves has helped them reach an old age, and the science suggests their instinct may be right.

Magical food combinations

It's not just food and wine that have a synergy; as evident from the blue zones, so too do different combinations of foods. In Nicoya, they're famous for eating ingredients they call the "three sisters": beans, corn and squash. When eaten together, they provide an ideal hit of amino acids, as well as fibre, polyphenols and nutrients.

Other ingredients offer different health benefits. Cooking tomatoes in olive oil makes it easier for us to absorb lycopene, the phytochemical in the fruit that gives them their red colour. Lycopene has powerful antioxidant properties, which may boost our brain health and help fight cancer.

Similarly, drizzling olive oil on veggies will increase the bioavailability of the nutrients. This is because they're fat-soluble and olive oil is, of course, a fat.

An interesting example is a simple base for dishes that is used in one way or another around the world. In France, they call it *mirepoix*, in Italy, *soffritto*, in the United States, the holy trinity, and in Poland, *włoszczyzna*, which literally translates to "Italian stuff". The ingredients vary slightly depending on where it's made, but it's commonly onion, celery and carrot, finely diced and cooked down slowly in olive oil. They are all healthy ingredients on their own, but when combined and cooked in oil they interact and become even more beneficial.

One study in 2009 gave healthy men a single serving of *sofritto* (the Spanish version made with onions, olive oil, tomatoes and salt) and found that their inflammatory biomarkers had improved when tested 24 hours later. "The preparation of *sofrito* modifies the bioactive compounds (carotenoids and polyphenols) in the ingredients to more bioavailable forms, promoting cis-lycopene formation and polyphenol bioaccessibility," explained the study. "The positive health effects of this tomato-based product may be attributed not only to lycopene, but to the bioactive compounds of all the ingredients."[110]

To me, this makes sense on an instinctive level, simply because these ingredients taste great together. We all know wine and food taste amazing together, each element acting on the other to improve it, so much so that there are professionals whose job is to find the perfect pairings. Cooked tomatoes are always tasty – raw ones can be hit or miss – and different cuisines around the world have been making their version of the *sofritto* for soups, stews, pasta dishes and pies for centuries.

Vinegar on the British classic, fish and chips, is another nutritionally clever combo, which doesn't just taste great but also helps you blunt the blood sugar spike you'd get from the carbohydrates.[111]

Why counting calories is a waste of time

People in the blue zones don't count calories – which is no surprise, since our utter fixation on doing so isn't conducive to a happy diet. There are a number of problems with basing our dietary choices on calorie-counting. For starters, the number of calories listed on the packet or thrown up by a Google search might not equate to the energy your body extracts from the food.

This was proven in a 2012 study by the US Department of Agriculture, in which scientists compared how much energy participants extracted from almonds with the number of calories attributed to them. The people absorbed an average of 4.6 calories per gram from the almonds, even though they were purported to have 6.1 calories per gram, a significant discrepancy of 32 per cent.[112] Not only this, but when the researchers compared individuals, they found the actual calories absorbed ranged from 2 per gram to 6 per gram. So, almonds for me are not the same as almonds for you, whatever the packet says.

Calories are not made equal

More pertinently still, the practice of calorie-counting is problematic due to its complete disregard of food's nutritional value. While there may be health benefits to be gained from eating less or periods of fasting, *what* you eat is crucial.

Dr Giles Yeo, whom we met in Part 1, has a lot to say about this; in fact, he wrote an entire book on it entitled *Why Calories Don't Count*. Over our Middle Eastern lunch in Cambridge, he explained his beef with calories. "If you're eating one particular type of food, of course calories count as a measure of the amount: 200g of chips is twice the portion of 100g of chips. If I eat 250 calories' worth of chips instead of 500 calories, of course I'll lose weight."

The problem arises when you're not comparing like with like – 100 calories of celery, for example, is not the same as 100 calories of Doritos. The "caloric availability" of the food depends hugely on what it is, Giles explains. Your body has to exert more effort to extract the calories from some foods than from others and this is not factored into calorie counts. "For example, for every 100 calories of protein we eat, we only absorb 70 calories. Fat, on the other hand, is nearly 100 per cent calorically available and carbohydrates can differ from 90 to 95 per cent available, depending on whether you're consuming a complex carb or sugar."

Caloric availability tends to be reduced by the protein content and fibre content of the food, which, as Giles says, is generally a marker of quality. UPFs tend to be lower in protein and fibre and therefore more calorically available, which means that if you eat 400 calories of them, it's likely that's what you'll get. Understanding that calorie-counting is a blunt tool and focusing instead on the quality of food is a better way to avoid putting on weight.

For me, the idea of calorie-counting is not only a futile exercise but also a joyless one. As Giles says, there's no consideration for the nutritional value or the taste. Counting calories makes eating feel like a dry, transactional process where nothing else matters but the numbers on a page. Food is not maths and nor should it be. If you're going to change your diet, and you want long-term effects from it, you need to eat things you find tasty and satisfying. This is one of the most critical aspects of longevity diets – they make their food taste good.

The complete absence of UPFs

In the traditional diets of all the blue zones, everything was homemade. UPFs simply did not exist. Times have changed and now, of course, they have access to these products. But the elderly populations there, who've made it to 90 and 100, have spent a lifetime not eating them.

No links between UPFs and positive health outcomes

Earlier we learnt what UPFs are, so now let's look at what they do. A growing body of evidence is showing that dietary exposure to UPFs is associated with at least one negative health outcome; these include cancer, obesity, cardiometabolic risk, irritable bowel syndrome, depression, frailty and what scientists call "all-cause mortality", which in human-speak means death. No study has found an association between UPFs and positive health outcomes.[113]

We don't really need a scientist to tell us this. It's something we know instinctively. Think about it for a second. How do these two different things make you feel: your mum's homemade lasagne, burnished, bubbling and crispy with lashings of creamy bechamel in between the luscious pasta layers, compared to, ding, your microwave lasagne is ready: wet, soggy, small, soft, sugary and over before you can spell it.

We evangelise about the power of a good home-cooked

meal. It's associated with warmth, comfort, satisfaction, wellbeing, good health and even the ability to remedy illness. Chicken soup is the most powerful example of this. Spain, America, Portugal, Italy, Romania, Moldova, Algeria, Vietnam, the Philippines, Poland, Greece, Colombia, Georgia, Peru, Mexico and South Korea all have their own versions of it and all attach soothing, healing qualities to it, recommending it for everything from colds and fevers to hangovers.

Other recipes give us the same nourishing feeling. Flavoursome stews of tender meat and root vegetables that have soaked up all the sauce; warm pasta bakes; flaky chicken pies with fresh steamed green veg and waxy new potatoes with melting salted butter – these dishes just feel good. UPFs have displaced these real foods, so much so that they now make up nearly 60 per cent of the calories we eat in the UK – a rate of consumption that's four times higher than Italy's – meaning the bulk of our diet, the predominant calorie source, is ultra-processed.[114]

UPFs and overeating

At first, researchers assumed it was the nutrient content of UPFs that was the problem, but then a curious study suggested otherwise. Kevin Hall, a senior investigator at the US National Institutes of Health, where he studies the regulation of body weight and metabolism, conducted an experiment in which he persuaded a group of 20 healthy volunteers to live in a laboratory for a month. Splitting them into two groups, he fed one a diet of UPFs and the other minimally processed foods for two-week periods and then switched them over. Both groups were told they could eat as much as they wanted and were given portions twice the size they'd need to maintain their body weight. Crucially, both diets were nutritionally matched, meaning the amounts of fat, sugar, salt, fibre, carbohydrates and protein were the same.

The results surprised even Dr Hall, who'd assumed, like others, that it was the fat, salt and sugar in UPFs that were important, not the way they were processed. During the two weeks of eating UPFs, the volunteers, on average, ate an extra 508 calories per day and put on a kilogram of weight in body fat. On the unprocessed diet, people ate less and lost weight. In other words, even though the food was matched nutritionally, and volunteers reported that the diets were equally tasty, something about the ultra-processed one was driving them to consume more.

"This is the first study to demonstrate that there is a causal relationship," Dr Hall told the BBC at the time in 2019. Previous studies had been observational (i.e. unable to show cause and effect). This had been the first randomised control trial, where a group of people are chosen at random to receive the "intervention", in this case UPFs, and another group, also chosen at random, acts as the "control" and is given a different intervention, a dummy intervention (a placebo) or nothing at all.[115]

"Ultra-processed foods led to increases in calorie intake and in body weight and in fat," said Hall.

But why is this the case? Why would UPFs make us overconsume even when they taste at best the same and in most cases worse than real food?

One theory Dr Hall has is that UPFs mess with our hunger hormones. When people ate the unprocessed diet their levels of PYY – a hormone that studies have shown reduces appetite – went up, even though they ate fewer calories than the other group, and their levels of the hunger hormone, ghrelin, went down.[116]

A novel set of substances

A few years ago, Dr Chris van Tulleken, an infectious diseases doctor and BBC broadcaster, decided to do a deep dive into what he calls our "new age of eating", in which "most of our calories come from an entirely novel set of substances". In 2023, he published the best-selling *Ultra Processed People: Why do we all eat stuff that isn't food … and why can't we stop?*, in which he charts the birth of UPFs, examines the studies investigating their impact on our health and makes them all sound very unappealing.

A key characteristic of UPFs is that they are both "soft" and "dry" at the same time, he says, which is troubling for our health. They're soft because they're foods that have been processed, broken down to such an enormous extent that the "food matrix" is destroyed, which can alter the way we absorb the energy and nutrients. Take, for example, a piece of corn on the cob: this can become sweetcorn in a can, or it can be broken down into cornmeal (polenta), or turned into corn starch (which is obtained by extracting the starch from the corn grain), and from there to modified maize (corn) starch, an ingredient now so commonplace in our foods you'd believe it was innocuous.

Modified starches, which include maize, are made by taking the extracted starch and altering it with chemical compounds. "Thin your starch with acid, and it's useful for textiles and laundry," writes Dr van Tulleken. "Treat it with propylene oxide, and you get that gloopy feel for salad dressings. Mix it with phosphoric acid, and you can improve stability through multiple cycles of freezing and thawing – perfect for pie fillings. And maltodextrins (short glucose polymers – a form of modified starch) can do things like giving a surface sheen and creaminess to what people think is a "milkshake". No more need for expensive dairy fats: these starches come from crops that can be grown at vast scales and at a fraction of the cost."

In short, UPFs are chemically altered foods, broken down and reconstructed to form items that resemble real foods. They are so soft that you have to do much less chewing to eat them and can therefore consume them a lot faster, which means you can take in more calories per minute and not realise you're full for some time.

They're "dry" because they tend to have the water removed from them to improve their shelf-life, which normally means they contain more calories per bite, so not only are you able to eat them fast, you're also taking in calorie-dense food at speed. Unlike calorie-dense whole foods, such as nuts, these foods are in most cases void of any nutritional value.[117]

Plus, modified starch is not tasty; it's just an odourless, tasteless white power, so additives – things like flavourings, artificial sweeteners, colours, emulsifiers and preservatives – have to be used to make the finished result palatable. Several studies have shown that these additives might be linked to inflammation and metabolic disease and could have a negative impact on our gut microbiome, which in turn could be detrimental to brain health.[118]

Weight gain, anxiety and brain changes

When Dr van Tulleken used himself as a guinea pig, eating a diet that was 80 per cent ultra-processed for an entire month, the effects were brutal. He gained 7kg, going from a healthy weight to overweight, had piles from constipation and experienced insomnia, anxiety, sluggishness and heartburn. "I felt 10 years older," he told the BBC.[119]

He became disgusted by the food but also felt a compulsion to keep eating it. Scarily, in just four weeks, scans showed that the areas in his brain responsible for reward had linked up with those associated with repetitive and automatic behaviours. "Eating ultra-processed food became something my brain simply told me to do, without me even wanting it," he said. Although he didn't like it, he was finding it hard to stop, in a similar way that a smoker struggles to give up cigarettes, even though the desire to do so is there.

Grape juice concentrate and aggressive marketing

A big problem with UPFs is that it can be very hard for the consumer to understand the labels. Hattie Burt is senior policy and international projects officer at Action on Sugar, a research and advocacy group working to reduce sugar consumption in the UK. "Many of the products aimed at children have scary amounts of sugar in them and often the sugar comes from things like grape juice concentrate, which to any conscientious parent checking the back of the packet sounds healthy."

> This is misleading, she says, and made even more so by the common addition of health claims such as "no added sugar". In the UK, this label simply means that no free sugars, such as table sugar, have been added, but naturally occurring sugars like those found in juice concentrate may have been. "There's misinformation around things like honey, coconut sugar and other things that sound like they should be healthier. They are just free sugars in exactly the same way."
>
> She thinks that part of the reason for our high consumption of UPFs in the UK is the way it's constantly advertised to us. "A third of food advertising in the UK goes towards confectionery, snacks, desserts and soft drinks," says Hattie. "One per cent is on fruit and vegetables. When you think about the adverts you see they're not for mushrooms and carrots, are they? All these adverts are directing us to buy and consume more processed food products that are cheap for the manufacturer to make and much more profitable than fruit and veg."

Tampering with the way the brain perceives food

There is another fascinating theory behind why UPFs are doing us harm: it's known as nutritional mismatch. It's the idea that if what we taste – sugar, for example – doesn't match the calories or nutrients we receive from a food or drink, it can throw off our metabolism and confuse our brain.[120]

In 2020 a neuroscientist called Dana Small at Yale University decided to investigate how artificially sweetened drinks affect the brain and gut. She ran experiments using drinks that were equally sweet but contained different amounts of calories and found that it was the drink that was nutritionally matched that caused the appropriate metabolic response and the biggest spike in brain activity.[121] Chris van Tulleken suspects the idea of nutritional mismatch might extend beyond sugar – a packet of crisps might taste very umami but then never deliver the protein hit our internal physiology might expect, which could lead us to continue eating in the naive hope of finding these missing nutrients.[122]

It's also a subject that Mark Schatzker, a Canadian author, has written at length about in his two books, *The Dorito Effect* and *The End of Craving*.

In the latter he writes: "For as long as humans and their ancestors have existed, the taste of a calorie matched the energy it delivered. In the span of just a few decades, that has changed. Calories don't 'mean' what they used to. We have tampered with the very way the brain perceives food. This is what has set so many of us on a path to weight gain. We changed food, and it changed us."[123]

He believes this is a crucial reason behind the obesity crises that are affecting most of the world.

Inevitably, as the modern world encroaches, the blue zones are seeing an influx of UPFs that didn't exist in the diets of those who've reached the age of 100. In fact, the traditional diets of those areas are under threat and even at risk of dying out in some places. This is the fear of Dan Buettner, the National Geographic writer who's built his career on exploring and documenting the blue zones. Speaking to me via video-call from his sunny home in Miami, he said: "In every one of the blue zones they want to be modern too. They're subject to the same advertising as we are and develop a taste for these processed, junk, fast foods. Their old diet goes by the wayside, and we can see very clearly that as it does, so too does their longevity."

How does it feel to watch these strong traditional diets in places where he's spent so much time become diluted by Western habits? "It's like watching the slow death of somebody you love," he says gravely.

Gut feelings

Perhaps the key to the good health of the blue-zoners lies in their guts. All five regions – whether they're aware of it or not – eat very gut-healthy diets.

Our guts are home to 100 trillion microbes – a mix of bacteria, archaea, fungi and viruses – an ecosystem that is collectively known as the gut microbiome. It weighs around 2kg, which is heavier than the average human brain, and science is only just beginning to understand its critical importance to our health – in fact, it's only in the last 15 years that key findings have been made.

Put simply, we have both good and bad microbes that, as one scientific review puts it, "have tremendous potential to impact our physiology, both in health and in disease. They contribute to metabolic functions, protect against pathogens, educate the immune system, and, through these basic functions, affect directly or indirectly most of our physiological functions."[124] Indeed, our gut microbiome has such an influence that it's often referred to as the "second brain", working in conjunction with the one in our head.

Half bacteria, half human

I wanted to know more about this hidden world, so I called up a neighbour of mine and invited her to a local bakery for a chocolate bun and a chat about guts.

Dr Emily Leeming, is, in her own words, a "gut microbiome nerd", but she began her career doing something quite different: working as a private chef for the rich and famous on superyachts in the Caribbean Sea. There, she encountered many people on extreme and restrictive diets who would profess their supposed health benefits, but Emily was less than convinced. Having studied nutrition at university, and finding that she missed science, she returned to the UK to discover the truth about how food affects our health, focusing her PhD and following career on the gut microbiome.

"We would die without our microbes," explains Emily, as we bite into just-baked buns filled with chocolate custard. "When mice have them removed in experiments, they become withdrawn, antisocial and quickly die."

We have co-evolved with our microbes and now have a dynamic relationship with them. "We're half bacteria, half human," says Emily. "If aliens came down from space they wouldn't say we were a human species but a hybrid species. Looking after the ecosystem of microbes that live in our gut is really looking after ourselves."

While other factors such as sleep, stress, exercise and antibiotic use can affect our gut microbiome, the main influence on it is what we eat. Each of us has the means to alter our internal ecosystems, influencing the levels and types of good bacteria in them. We can foster a gang, a whole community of good guys, which will, in turn, improve both our physical and mental health.

More excitingly still, is that it doesn't take years to see the results. Some research suggests that it only takes a matter of days to change the make-up of our gut microbiome, with modifications to our diet.[125]

So, what would the critters like on the menu?

Fibre and polyphenols

Like us, our microbes have food preferences. But what the "good guys", or helpful bacteria, and the "bad guys", or unhelpful bacteria, like is quite different.

Because this is an emerging field of study, scientists are still learning what foods work best and to what extent this differs from person to person – my good gut bacteria may like apples whereas yours may want tofu – but what we can say for sure is that fibre is a winner and an easy place to start.

"Our gut microbiome has a field day when we eat fibre," says Emily. "It throws a party." This is why legumes are a brilliant food category to add to your diet; they feed our microbes as well as us. As we know, the blue zones all love legumes.

Current guidelines recommend adults eat 30g of fibre per day, but most of us only manage 20g maximum. Emily thinks this could be due to fibre's unglamorous reputation. "We have this big taboo about poo and fibre is associated with it – known for helping to make you go."

It's time to forget that and get our fill of fibre, because it feeds our gut, and our gut has such an enormous impact on our health. "Every 7g increase of fibre in our diets reduces our risk of heart disease, type 2 diabetes and stroke by 6–7 per cent," says Emily.

It doesn't mean laboriously chewing our way through heaps of raw kale, as one might imagine. Instead, Emily recommends homing in on the foods that have the highest fibre content. "Legumes, for example, are much higher in fibre than most fruits and vegetables," says Emily. Lentils, kidney beans and split peas are particularly good choices as they have 10.7g, 7.4g and 8.3g of fibre per 100g respectively, whereas most vegetables typically have only 2–4g per 100g.[126]

The plant-centred diet in the blue zones, with a particular emphasis on legumes, means they not only eat plenty of fibre; they also get a good dose of polyphenols, the beneficial plant chemicals we learnt about earlier.

Polyphenols have a positive effect on the gut, possibly stimulating the growth of good bacteria and blocking the growth of bad.[127,128] Among the most polyphenol-rich foods are olives and olive oil; nuts and seeds, particularly chestnuts – favoured in Sardinia – as well as pecans, almonds and hazelnuts; red wine; dark chocolate; legumes; tofu; and vegetables, in particular red and green chicory, red onion, artichokes and spinach.[129]

Gut diversity

It seems that our guts also enjoy diversity. And there is evidence to suggest that eating a variety of different plants fosters a healthy – i.e. diverse – gut microbiome.[130] The blue-zoners achieve this effortlessly by eating what's available seasonally, thereby consuming a wide range of different plants throughout the year.

They also help their gut diversity by eating fermented foods, such as the yoghurt enjoyed in Sardinia and Ikaria. A study by Stanford School of Medicine found that a diet rich in fermented foods increases the diversity of our gut microbes and decreases signs of inflammation.[131]

Other research shows that a more diverse gut microbiome is a more resilient one that functions better and keeps us healthier than a gut with fewer species of microbes.[132] In a clinical trial, 36 healthy adults were randomly assigned either a 10-week diet of fermented foods such as yoghurt, kefir, fermented cottage cheese, kimchi (and other fermented vegetables), vegetable brine drinks and kombucha tea, or a diet high in fibre comprised of vegetables, nuts, seeds, whole grains, fruit and legumes. Interestingly, only in the fermented group did microbial diversity increase and signs of inflammation decrease.

Dr Justin Sonnenburg called it a "stunning finding" and said: "It provides one of the first examples of how a simple change in diet can reproducibly remodel the microbiota across a cohort of healthy adults".[133] In other words, if you want to change the make-up of your gut microbiome, you can.

Happy meals? The gut's role in our mental health

Can food make you happy? If I was the one being asked this question I wouldn't hesitate. Of course it can, I'd say, with the kind of unwavering certainty an Italian zia displays when asked if her cooking is better than Maria's down the road.

I'd think of comfort food, the very purpose of which is to lift our spirits. It makes us feel good, it cheers us up, it softens a bad day. And it's interesting because while we'd all select a different dish to fulfil this role, these choices tend to follow the same broad themes: carbohydrate-rich, saucy, unpretentious, home-cooked and nearly always nostalgic. If you want to make someone happy, find out what their favourite food was growing up and cook them something that has echoes of it. This is because food is so linked to memory. Potatoes cut and fried in a certain way aren't just potatoes, they're a portal to somewhere else, as transportive, in my view, as music. A song can take you somewhere and so can food.

Lots of types of food make me happy: thick Greek yoghurt with perfect summer blackberries, the ones that are sweet and juicy but also requisitely tart; carbonara made with the super-fresh yellow-yolked eggs from the lady who has chickens across the road from Mum's; dark, bitter chocolate with unexpected salt crystals; savoury pies from literally every cuisine, including multi-layered filo pastry burek filled with cheese, spinach, leek or pumpkin eaten across the Balkans and Turkey; a Cornish pasty with thick, stodgy shortcrust pastry and classic beef, potato and swede filling; and – *God bless Scotland* – the macaroni pie, a hot-water-crust pastry case filled with delicious macaroni cheese. Pasta and pastry in a loving union? The world is good.

But can food affect your mood more than just transiently? Can it bring about longer-term changes to how you feel? Scientists are starting to think so.

The standout study on the link between diet and mental wellbeing comes from Australia and a woman people call the "mother of nutritional psychiatry", Professor Felice Jacka. In a randomised controlled trial of participants with depression she conducted in 2017, one group was given help from a nutritionist to adopt a Mediterranean-style diet, while the other was given social support but instructed to stick to their normal diet.

After three months, the group on the Med diet experienced a much greater reduction in their depressive symptoms than the other group, with a third meeting the criteria for remission, compared to 8 per cent in the other group.[134] "These results were not explained by changes in physical activity or body weight, but were closely related to the extent of dietary change," according to the study. "In other words, those who improved their diet the most experienced the greatest benefit to their depression."[135]

The Med diet, known for its emphasis on unprocessed, plant foods, healthy protein and fat, is "consistently associated with better mental health outcomes," says Professor Jacka.

"These diets are also high in fibre, which is essential for gut microbiota. We're increasingly understanding that the gut is really the driver of health, including mental health, so keeping fibre intake high through the consumption of plant foods is very important."[136]

The impact of a plant-based diet high in gut-friendly fibre on mental health had been seen before in observational studies. Another Australian study showed that the amount of fruit and vegetables a person ate could predict how happy and satisfied with life they were over a two-year period. An increase in consumption led to an increase in happiness.[137]

Why is this happening?

The thinking behind all this is that a healthy diet contributes to a healthy gut which, through something known as the gut–brain axis, can communicate with the brain, directly affecting the way we feel. The gut–brain axis is a pathway that allows bi-directional communication between the brain and the gut.

I put the question simply to Dr Emily Leeming, the gut-health expert: can food make us happy? "Yes, it can and more than we think. It's not temporary – i.e. *this tastes delicious and it's making me feel good right now* – it's actually a huge part of our health and wellbeing."

One of the reasons experts think this may be, Emily explains, is that the areas of the brain that are associated with emotional regulation (and can shrink in people with mood disorders) are the same as those that are seen to increase in size and function better when people eat a healthier diet.

Another is tryptophan. This is an amino acid derived from our diet that is also a key building block of serotonin (the neurotransmitter or hormone that makes us feel happy). Unlike serotonin, which is made in our gut but cannot cross the blood–brain barrier, tryptophan can because of its smaller size. "It's like buying a ready-made sofa," says Emily. "That's your serotonin. It's too big to get through the door. Tryptophan, on the other hand, is like an Ikea flat-pack. You get it through the door and then have to build it locally, on site, that is, in your brain. So your gut has huge involvement with your brain."

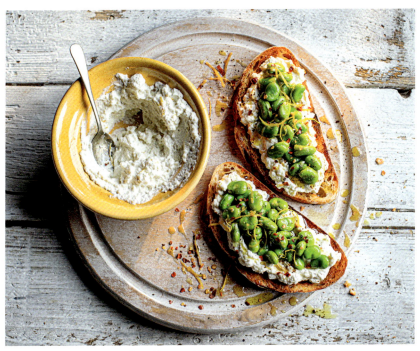

SPRING Broad beans with ricotta on sourdough (p166)

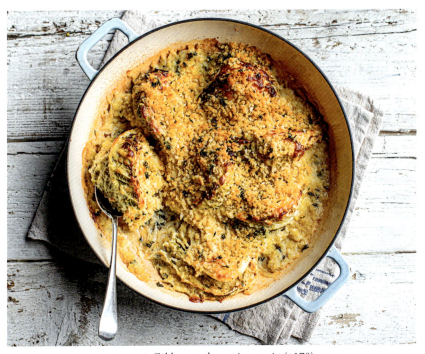

SPRING Cabbage and pecorino gratin (p170)

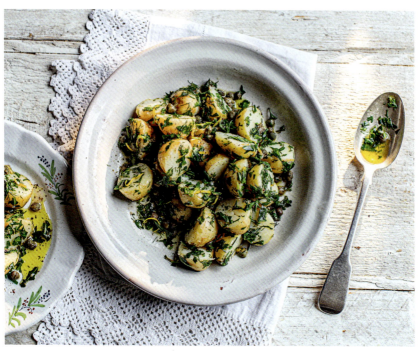

SPRING Warm potato salad with capers, dill and lemon (p177)

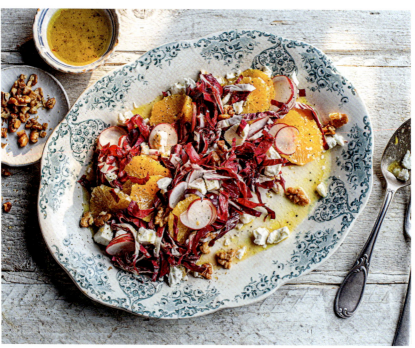

SPRING Radicchio, orange and feta salad with toasted walnuts (p169)

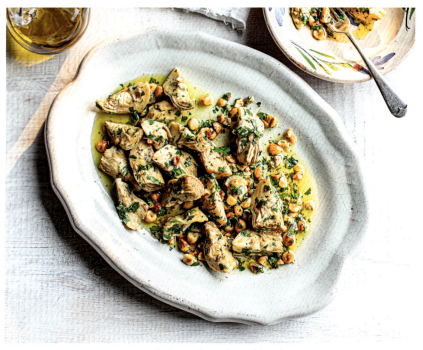

SUMMER Artichokes with parsley and hazelnuts (p180)

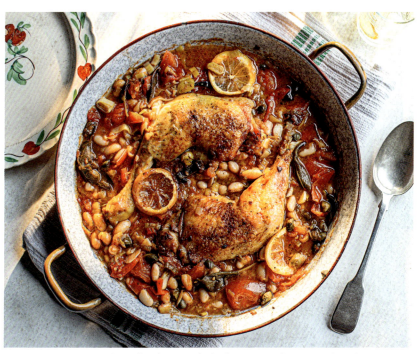

SUMMER Cannellini beans with chicken, sage and tomatoes (p189)

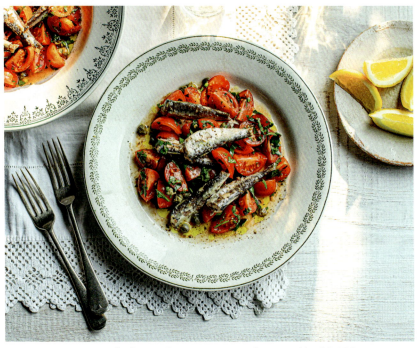
SUMMER Sardines with tomatoes, capers, lemon and basil (p188)

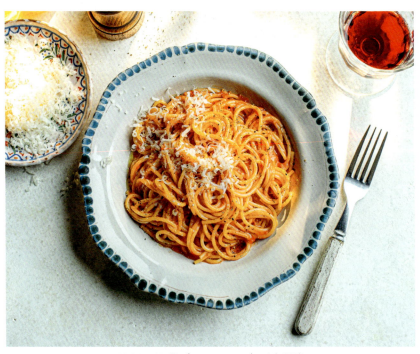
SUMMER Fresh tomato spaghetti (p192)

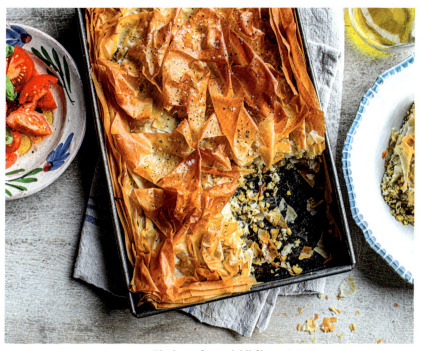

AUTUMN Chickpea, feta and dill filo pie (p198)

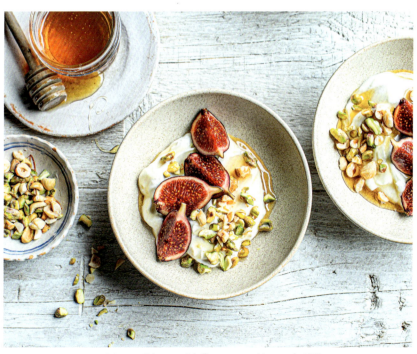

AUTUMN Ricotta with figs, nuts and honey (p205)

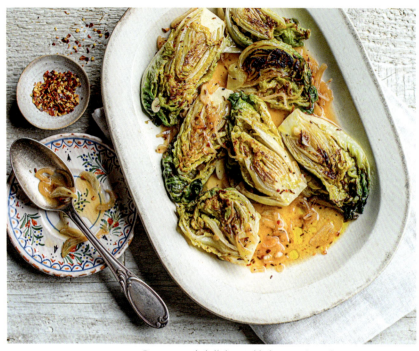

AUTUMN Caraway and chilli braised baby gem (p200)

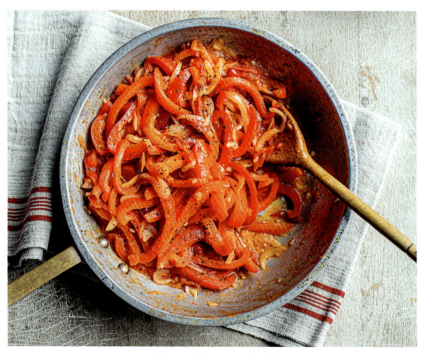

AUTUMN Peperonata (p197)

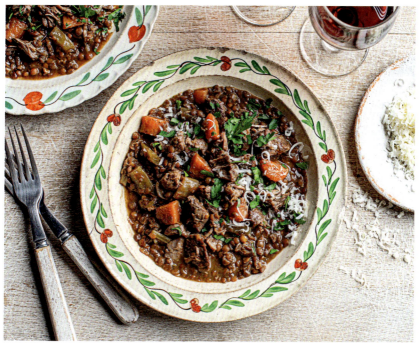

WINTER Slow-cooked beef with thyme, garlic and brown lentils (p230)

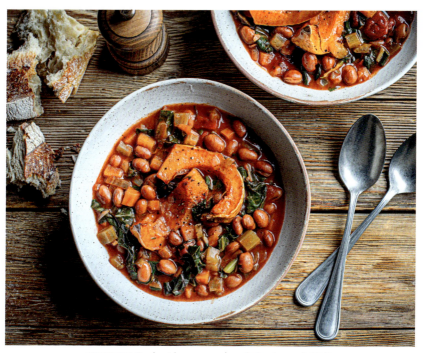

WINTER Borlotti bean, squash and chard stew (p224)

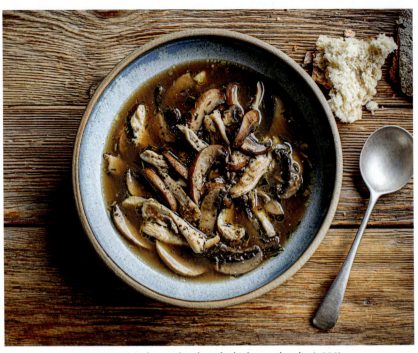

WINTER Mushroom broth with chicken and garlic (p222)

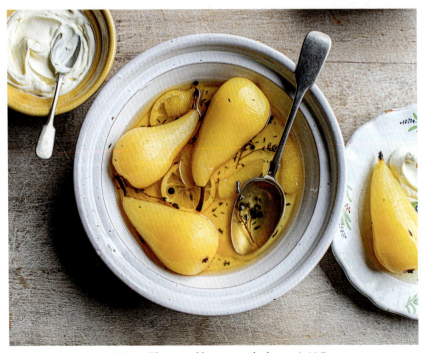

WINTER Thyme and lemon poached pears (p226)

The psychology of eating together

For a large chunk of my working life, I've eaten my main meal of the day alone. Being a writer whose office is her home, it was inevitable. My flatmate was at work and so around 1 or 2pm I'd sit down to lunch by myself. It was normally some variation of a salad with lots of different things in it, or pasta or a stir-fry when I could be bothered, and I'd eat it at the same place where I did my work, my kitchen table. To be fair, it was an improvement on how I used to eat lunch when working in the office of a national newspaper – miserably, from a plastic box with a plastic fork while staring at my screen and clicking the mouse occasionally, pretending I was still working. Sometimes I'd try to silently protest against this pointless and counter-productive culture of presenteeism by taking my lunch box to the canteen, a gloomy place starved of natural light or, when the weather was acceptable, a small park where I'd sit on a bench and munch my plastic-infused, cold food and watch curiously as other smartly dressed professionals did the same. These days I eat lunch most days with my partner – still at the kitchen table, but in a wholly better way. And when I look back on my former working-lunch routine I find it weird and sad.

Mealtimes and the anticipation of them were my favourite moments as a child; the kitchen full of smells, steam, noises, intrigue and excitement. I'd climb onto the side and sit and watch as my dad cooked dinner, studying carefully how he chopped onions and asking him why he added this ingredient and not that. When we sat down to eat as a family, we'd talk about the food in front of us and all the other random topics that a kid's developing mind is interested in. A lot of my education happened around the dinner table from the conversations we would have there.

We were lucky to go on holiday a lot when I was growing up, particularly to France, where I developed a deeper understanding of the world through food and eating communally. I wanted to eat exactly how my parents did, so even as a child I dug into *moules marinière* (the French dish of juicy, plump mussels in garlic and wine) as if they were a bowl of sweets; on one of those holidays I tasted a horizon-expanding pear ice cream that I've never forgotten, and on a boat in Italy one summer, I ate pasta with a tomato, tuna and parsley sauce that was so revelatory to me that, encouraged by my mum, I nervously went to give my compliments to the chef, who was so amused he gave me another adult-sized portion.

I was fortunate to have these experiences and I thank my parents for, consciously or not, making food such a focal pleasure in my life. Food, growing up, wasn't just about eating but in large part about sharing ideas and learning about culture. It was a communal, collaborative experience, one that was completely different from sitting alone on a park bench with a plastic lunch box.

Centenarians in longevity hotspots tend to have eaten communally all their lives and, just like their emphasis on vegetables, this is a vital part of their happy diet.

Warding off future weight problems

A lot of research has been done revealing the multitude of benefits that come from eating together at a table. Studies have been done on children showing that eating together at a table can improve their communication skills and their self-esteem and ward off weight problems in the future.[138] A 2015 study found a direct correlation between how often adolescents sat down for a family meal and their likelihood of weight or obesity problems 10 years later – unsurprisingly, the more communal meals, the better their outcome.[139] Another study suggested that family meals instil healthy eating habits in children and are associated with a better diet overall, with more fruit and vegetables and fewer sugary drinks.[140]

People who eat together have more friends

It's not just children who benefit, although I believe a positive association with food as a child will last a lifetime. Research from Oxford University's Experimental Psychology Department found that the more often people ate in company, the more likely they were to feel happy, be satisfied with their lives and to have close friends they could depend on for support. It also found them to be "more trusting" of others and more engaged with their local communities.[141]

Intrigued, I picked up the phone and gave the study's author, Professor Robin Dunbar, a call. "Neuro-imaging has shown that eating triggers the endorphin effect which gives you a sense of calmness, a sense of relaxation, a contentedness and plays a role in social bonding," he told me. "When you do so in company and in synchrony with somebody else it ramps up that endorphin effect." In essence, eating makes you feel good and eating together makes you feel even better, which in turn makes you feel more bonded to that person.

When you think about it, we've created a lot of rituals

around eating and drinking that synchronise these acts, Professor Dunbar said. "We regulate eating with courses and we propose toasts and buy rounds so everyone drinks together." The same is also true of other activities that release endorphins. Singing, dancing, laughing and even exercise will all produce more endorphins when done in company than alone.

"We first saw this effect years ago in an experiment using the university rowing team," he went on. Researchers observed the difference between the release of endorphins between the athletes doing solo exercise on rowing machines and when they exercised in tandem, with the machines connected to one another to form a virtual boat. "The endorphin effect was doubled. It's really quite extraordinary. And we now know exactly the same thing happens with eating. Eating will give you an endorphin hit but if you do it socially you get a much bigger hit and create this sense of bonding to the person or people you're sitting with."

Professor Dunbar thinks this is why people who eat in company more often have been shown to have more close friends or, as he calls them, "shoulders to cry on – people you'd go to in a crisis", because it is an act that helps people to connect with one another more easily.

His study showed that the communal meals that resulted in people feeling closest to those they dined with were in the evenings, rather than at lunch, because they tended to involve more people, more laughter, more reminiscing and alcohol.

Whether you eat with lots of people or just one and whether that's at a restaurant or at home, Professor Dunbar recommends doing it as much as you can. "It's not just important in maintaining your psychological health, but good for your physical health too, because endorphins trigger the release of natural killer cells, which target viruses and some cancers."

Professor Dunbar also referred to the huge amount of evidence from epidemiological studies showing that the quality and number of close friendships you have is one of the most reliable predictors of your future psychological and physical health and wellbeing and even of how long you will live. In case you're wondering, the optimum number is five and this number can include family members.

One last, curious fact: if you're after an even bigger hit of endorphins, try eating something spicy or astringent – it's probably the reason we love tea and coffee so much, according to Professor Dunbar (the astringency in them is due to tannins). When it comes to maintaining your relationships, it could be that a curry is better than a risotto.

Nutritional intelligence

Maybe you've heard of a practice called "intuitive eating". It's the notion of listening to your body's signals around food: how hungry you are, how full you are and trusting your intuition to make the right choices when it comes to what to eat. This may sound a little woo-woo, but it turns out the idea that humans intuitively select food based on nutritional needs may be rooted in science.

The theory has been shown in studies on both animals and children. A study from 2012 found that black howler monkeys selected foods high in the minerals they became deficient in after their normal food sources were disrupted by a hurricane.[142]

More fascinating still was a study back in 1939 by a researcher named Dr Clara Davis, who allowed just-weaned children to pick their own food and how much of it they wanted to eat over the course of six months to a year. The children lived in an orphanage and, in an experiment that wouldn't be allowed now, were presented every mealtime with a buffet of 34 foods, including orange juice, bone marrow, turnips, sour milk, peaches, liver, lamb, potatoes and a little bowl of salt, and ate what they wanted without any nudges or encouragement by nurses. It was Dr Davis's belief that, given the choice, the children would select for themselves a nutritious diet and the results bore this out. The kids often dined on rather odd combinations, such as liver and orange juice for breakfast or banana and eggs for dinner, but in general showed themselves to be omnivorous with changing tastes.

Sometimes they'd get a real taste for a certain ingredient and eat it over and over again for a while, something Dr Davis called "jags" – "egg jags", "meat jags". She couldn't conclude for definite why this occurred but suspected the waves of cravings aligned with what the children needed at that time for "optimal growth".[143]

One of the children, who began the experiment with rickets, chose both cod liver oil and milk containing cod liver oil from the buffet with each meal, which he drank voluntarily every day until his rickets was gone. By the end of the experiment, all the children had nourished themselves optimally and grown healthily. "They achieved the goal, by widely various means," Dr Davis said of the study. "There were no failures of infants to manage their own diets; all had hearty appetites; all throve."[144]

Positive cravings

If children can intuit a healthy diet, surely so too can adults? It's a question the Canadian author Mark Schatzker has spent time pondering and became so intrigued by that he partnered with a scientist at Bristol University, Professor Jeff Brunstrom, to run his own experiment on it. They showed 128 adults pictures of different pairings of fruit and vegetables and asked them which they preferred. After controlling for factors such as "explicit nutritional knowledge and food energy density", they observed a "significant tendency to select pairings that offered a greater total micronutrient intake and greater 'micronutrient complementarity', i.e. a broader range of micronutrients."

"We're referring to it as 'nutritional intelligence'," Mark says on a video-call from Toronto, Canada, where he lives. It's the theory that our dietary inclinations are informed in part by what our bodies need. "We're not just attracted to carbs, fat and protein; we're also attracted to foods that deliver particular vitamins and minerals."

On a purely anecdotal basis, I sometimes get cravings for seemingly random ingredients – for example, every now and then, vividly coloured beetroot might scream out to me from the supermarket shelf, an Alice in Wonderland "Eat Me" sign metaphorically above it. On other occasions, I get a yearning for cooked dark greens like spinach or cavolo nero and about once or twice a year I simply must eat a steak. I've always wondered whether these cravings represented more than just a desire for a certain flavour and were my body's way of directing me towards something I needed, like iron or potassium.

"Your desires can nourish you," says Mark, after I tell him my experience. "And it makes sense in the very simple sense that animals do it. They don't know what vitamin C or vitamin E is and yet they nourish themselves well."

In other words, we know what's good for us. Mark gives the example of fruit. "Really good fruit tastes good because it's filled with vitamins and minerals, not just sugar. What's interesting is that when fruit is ultra-sweet it's ultra-ripe and we don't like it like that, it doesn't taste good. When you look at an ultra-ripe fruit metabolically, at its antioxidant cycle, you can see that it's burned through all its vitamin C. I would say that's why we have this sense of taste, because you're deciding if something is *good*."

Mark hopes there will soon be more research in this field and is conducting more himself with Professor Brunstrom.

"Our appetite is not stupid," he says. "It's not this Stone Age greed, stuffing our face with anything. It possesses an intelligence we don't understand. When you bite into an apple or a strawberry or a piece of cheese, your brain is performing computation faster than we can imagine, based on all its previous experience of that food, and it's assigning it a value that I still think we don't even fully comprehend."

As outlined earlier in this part of the book, a potential problem for our nutritional wisdom or intelligence is nutritional mismatch – when flavour and nutrition don't match due to ultra-processing.

Mark believes that the fact that the sensory signals in our food environment have changed could be the root of our obesity crisis – our food today tells us "nutritional lies".

"We have artificial sweeteners and fake flavours. We have fat replacers, we put vitamins in our flour and our breakfast cereals. We put them in energy bars and candy bars. And it's created a food environment that our brain was not evolved to exist in. Our intelligence system has been led astray. And what these chaotic signals have created is what psychologists call uncertainty. The brain likes to predict, it wants to know what it's getting and one of the responses to uncertainty, which is very well known in psychology, is to want more." In other words, we overeat.

How to train your "second" brain

One theory suggests that our gut microbes play a role in our drive to eat certain things, both good and bad. They, as one paper puts it, are "under selective pressure to manipulate host eating behaviour to increase their fitness, sometimes at the expense of host fitness".[145]

For the avoidance of doubt, you are the host. It's a fascinating and vaguely spooky idea – that it's not really you making your food choices, but different microbial species vying for dominance in your gut. In order for them to thrive, they have to get you to eat what they want. In basic terms, if you regularly eat McDonalds, gut microbes that "specialise" in McDonalds will thrive and in turn, drive you to continue eating McDonalds.

Conversely, if you eat a lot of seaweed, as is common in Japan, you will develop microbes that thrive on seaweed. Thus, through their link to your brain, your microbes can alter your eating behaviour. This suggests that the more "healthy" food you eat, the more you'll want to eat and vice versa.

With all this in mind, the paper hypothesises that a higher diversity of species within your gut could be protective. This is because different species of microbes are competitive and the more you have, the more they will fight among themselves for "resources". "A less diverse microbial population is likely to have species within it that have large population sizes and more resources available for host manipulation. Moreover, the larger a particular microbial population is, the more power it would have to manipulate the host."

The best way to diversify your gut, as we saw earlier, is to diversify your diet. Add, add, add – new plants, a range of nuts and seeds, fruits you don't normally eat, different fermented foods, a rainbow of vegetables.

Perhaps this is the real meaning of "nutritional intelligence". A positive feedback loop between "us" and our gut microbes.

Food at the heart of a nourishing lifestyle

Ageing well is a puzzle and diet is one piece of that puzzle. It's a big piece, the one right in the middle, but there are other pieces scattered around the edges that we must include to complete the picture.

A person who's spent her career investigating the factors that contribute to healthy ageing is Professor Rose Anne Kenny, a practising doctor, researcher and founding principal investigator of the Irish Longitudinal Study on Ageing, or TILDA, which was set up 15 years ago.

"There are two ways of looking at ageing," she says. "Chronological age, which is the number of candles on the birthday cake, and biological age, which is how old your cells are – we have a number of hallmarks, measures, that can tell us this. All cells age eventually but they age at different paces and when there's a lot of cell ageing that's when disease starts to happen. By understanding biological ageing and the triggers for it, we can intervene and slow down ageing on a cellular level."

As I mentioned at the beginning of this book, we all have a huge ability to influence our outcomes. Longevity is 80 per cent lifestyle factors and only 20 per cent genes. I also mentioned that there is no one thing that explains the blue-zoners' happy, healthy longevity; diet is key, but there is a whole web of factors alongside this, which are also increasingly backed up by fascinating new science.

Social connection and a sense of purpose

One of those lifestyle factors is friendship. Its inverse, loneliness, can be deadly, says Professor Kenny, causing us to age faster and die sooner. "Let me give you an example from a study done on monkeys," she said. "They are gregarious animals, as we are, but in this experiment a number of monkeys were isolated. After 48 hours, biopsies of the lymph nodes in the neck were taken – these are the glands that govern our immune response, our inflammatory response. Even within two days, the monkeys had started to have an inflammatory response – they recognised the loneliness as a toxic thing to the body and were treating it as if it were an infection. The fact that the body has an inflammatory response when we really do get an infection is obviously a good thing, and what we need, but if our body is responding to an infection that isn't there, that is not good for our biology."

The same biomarkers are seen in humans. "Loneliness triggers disease and people who are very lonely die earlier," says Professor Kenny. "We have evolved to need each other, to be part of a community and to engage face to face."

All the blue zones have strong communities and put a lot of emphasis on family. Their social set-up is quite different from ours in the UK. While it is common in the UK to relocate for work, people in the blue zones have traditionally lived and died in the place where they were born. This means the family unit and wider community have tended to stay together rather than scatter across the country. I see this with both my Sardinian and my Campanian families, where generations old and young live together in tight-knit units. Great-grandmothers help to look after their great-grandchildren.

My nonna died before her siblings, who are still alive today. Zia Filomena, the eldest, is 94 and still going strong – in fact, she is a central, revered and influential member of the community in her village in Italy. My mum has a sad theory: that if nonna and grandad had moved back to Italy or Sardinia instead of breaking the mould by deciding to live in the UK, then they both would have lived longer. By moving – an act considered quite rebellious by their peers at the time – they forged a completely different life for their family, affording each coming generation opportunities they might not otherwise have had, and I am very grateful to them, but there is no doubt that they sacrificed the comforting bosom of community to do so.

As my zia Filomena (great-aunt Phil) brilliantly demonstrates, it is uncommon for people in the blue zones to be isolated or disengaged from society. Everyone has a role to play, which brings us to another key, health-promoting factor: having a sense of purpose.

"Having a meaning to each day is important," says Professor Kenny. We're not talking here about being driven to change the world, or to maintain a high-flying job. Purpose can comprise small tasks – taking the bins out, doing the laundry, checking in on Tony across the road, baking your friend a cake, sending some emails – but consolidating them each morning is helpful.

"We haven't evolved to be good at drifting, to not have a purpose for the day." In the blue zones, they recognise this and even have sayings for it. In Nicoya, they call it "plan de vida" – their reason for waking up in the morning; and in Japan they talk about discovering their "ikigai", a pursuit that you're good at, you love, you can be paid for and the world needs.

Moving naturally

The people of the blue zones also exercise regularly which is critical for health. They don't have gym memberships, go jogging or sign up to Pilates classes – they walk, they garden, they do household chores. In the mountainous Nuoro region in Sardinia, everyone has to go up and down steep hills just to fulfil their daily tasks – buy bread, go to church. Natural movement is incorporated into their days, so they're getting exercise without it being a conscious effort. Of all the blue-zoners, only the Seventh-Day Adventists of Loma

Linda actively work at keeping fit, exercising intentionally like we do in the UK; nevertheless, instead of going for a lonely run or workout session, they tend to take part in community exercise classes with friends, which means they are socialising as well.

The key thing, as Professor Kenny says, is that they are moving a lot. "Sitting for long periods of time is not good for the brain. Standing up every 45 minutes wakes up the autonomic nervous system, which pumps blood around the systems and is very important for getting rid of toxins."

This is something we need to be more mindful of in our sedentary, screen-fixed lives. "Both anaerobic and aerobic are beneficial, and weight training and balance training are particularly beneficial over the age of 40," explains Professor Kenny. But we can also do ourselves much good simply by undertaking the sort of normal daily tasks that modernity is increasingly phasing out. This could be carrying the shopping rather than getting it delivered; taking the stairs rather than the lift; or simply walking more – much better than waiting for a bus!

Lack of stress

De-stressing rituals, of which exercise may be one for you, are also helpful. Being stressed pushes us into "fight or flight" mode – a physiological reaction that happens when we are faced with any sort of threat – but being in that mode when we don't need to be is not good for us, once again leading to inflammation. Practices like deep-breathing, meditation, mindfulness and yoga are brilliant for de-stressing.

Super-agers, like Vincenza Celea, our 97-year-old from

Molochio, know on an intuitive level what has kept them well. "I've always led a peaceful life, minimising stress," she said. "The pursuit of tranquillity is important for longevity. Stay active, work, enjoy family and always be kind. Good humour and prayer have helped me live a long life."

Another village resident, Assunta Longo, 91, who lost her partner 35 years ago, had this advice: "Live calmly, have a clear conscience and avoid a stressful and hectic life. Despite family sorrows, I am content with my life. We thank God for reaching this age."

Professor Kenny identifies sleeping well, being satisfied with your sex life (whatever that means for you), cold water exposure and creativity as other important lifestyle factors for slowing down the process of ageing. "There's some lovely science behind creativity," she says. "It suppresses the fight or flight component of the nervous system and enhances the 'parasympathetic' system – our rest and digest response." Doing something creative can also give you a sense of purpose; it can involve socialising and it can act as a form of mindfulness.

Where, I ask, does she place diet in terms of importance? "Very high. It's critical. I can't put one at the top of the tree but if I had to choose three, I'd say diet, friendship and exercise."

In other words, a holistic approach to health. Factors are interconnected and one can lead to another to create a nourishing lifestyle. In the blue zones, food and cooking are at the heart of life, giving a sense of purpose, strengthening relationships, requiring exercise, providing a way to de-stress and an outlet for creativity.

Angelo Matarozzo, 95, is living evidence of the benefits

of this approach: "Work, fresh air, genuine relationships and staying active contributed to my wellbeing. Long walks with friends to the mountains, picking mushrooms and returning on foot rejuvenated me. If you want to live long and healthily, be responsible and generous, hold onto values, and keep moving forward despite the challenges of modern life."

"One of the most important things to remember is how good quality of life gets after the age of 50," says Professor Kenny. "It's remarkable how much it improves. Everybody's assumption is that as you get older, life gets worse. But consistently ours and other studies have shown that life gets better after 50 and peaks around 78 or 80. You're wiser, you don't care as much what people think, your friendships are more solid and you don't have as many problems as when you're in your thirties or forties. When you're older you have more inner peace.

"The only reason quality of life starts to decline at 80 is because of physical illness. If you can manage physical illness, you will have happy ageing."

In this modern world, life can feel overwhelming, and health and happiness can seem like abstract concepts that are hard to grasp. There's no panacea that will fix everything, but going back to basics and focusing on something that is tangible but also a daily source of joy seems a very good place to start. With that being said, what's for lunch?

4

Five steps to a happier diet

So, here we are at the end of our culinary journey. What have we learnt, what conclusions can we draw, and how can we begin to shift our diet and eating habits into a happier gear?

As we have seen, good nutrition doesn't have to be complicated; in fact, people in the blue zones achieve it without trying. It's easy for them because it is just the way they live. You can make it easy for yourself, too, by repositioning eating well as a joyful part of your life, rather than an irksome duty, or some short-term dietary challenge.

If that's something you'd like to do, then here are five steps that will help you do it. Cheers to happy eating.

1. Put flavour first

Not until relatively late in my life did I ever hear anyone talk about food as if it were a bad thing – something to be feared, controlled, restricted or divided into moral and immoral camps. Though everybody in my family loves food, it was from my nonna that I took my biggest culinary inspiration, and it wouldn't have crossed her mind to consider food an enemy. I doubt we would have been able to explain the concept to her. Of course, she had the sense that eating 65 Maltesers might make your tummy hurt but the idea of demonising everyday ingredients such as bread or pasta or endowing magical properties on kale or blueberries would have seemed strange and certainly a waste of one's time. If I told her, for example, that some people avoid all carbs because they see them as "unhealthy", she would have said "rubbish" in her strong Italian accent and got back to the important business of encouraging me to eat: "*mangia, mangia*" – the instructive catchphrase of all Italian grandmothers.

For Nonna, if food was to be divided it was thus: good taste and bad taste. She didn't think about whether something was particularly "healthy"; she thought about the quality of the ingredients, the balance of tastes and the pleasingness of the texture.

This is the most important factor in eating to live to 100: flavour must come first. When flavour and nutrition are aligned, everything is simpler. You're not "going on a diet", there's no need for maintenance or control. The people of these longevity hotspots have eaten this way their entire lives; enjoying food and good nutrition in unconscious harmony. They do it by ensuring that everything they cook is delicious.

The genius of "cucina povera"

A lot of this interplay between good nutrition and good taste comes from the ingenuity of peasant food, which in Italy is known as "cucina povera" or the cuisine of the poor. All the blue zones, except Loma Linda, have peasant food cuisines, in which clever cooks had to work with what was available to make things taste good. I wanted to speak to somebody who had a deep understanding of this, somebody who lives and breathes this philosophy.

So I video-called the biggest flavour enthusiast I know, Italian chef Gennaro Contaldo, and caught him as he was cooking his lunch.

Gennaro, 74, is famous for his many cookbooks on Italian food, his TV show, *Two Greedy Italians*, and for being a mentor to British chef Jamie Oliver.

He picks up the call and immediately flips his camera to show me a pan of fennel, onions and cherry tomatoes simmering softly. Though he's lived in England now for many years, he still cooks in the way he learnt growing up in the seaside village of Minori, on Italy's Amalfi coast.

"We used to make fantastic dishes out of very little," he says, "taking what was in season and making the best of it."

Gennaro's mother and grandmother would find clever ways to maximise flavour and avoid waste, using what would otherwise be discarded fish heads to make wonderful soups or flavouring the *minestra maritata*, a nutritious soup packed with greens, with leftover bits of chicken or salami to add depth and umami. "We'd never chuck anything away, nothing at all," remembers Gennaro. "Throw away bread? You've got to be joking me. We'd dry it in the sun for two or three days and make bruschetta, breadcrumbs or a lovely bread salad."

You see the same thing in all the blue zones – there is a resourcefulness to the cooking; massive flavour is achieved with not a lot, and sorry-looking leftovers are transformed into the most wonderful dishes. No matter what they're making, good flavour is a priority.

Gennaro fell in love with flavour at a young age, picking herbs for his mother to use in her cooking. "Everything was fresh," he remembers of the local produce in Minori. "Vegetables had to be *crisp*. Where I come from, 'old' meant one day." He remembers going hunting with his father and grandfather (who lived to be 96 and 98 respectively). These early experiences taught him about the provenance of food, the quality of ingredients, the meaning of real flavour and in many ways nutrition. "We learnt about diet, the way to eat, without even realising that we were learning and mostly it was through the respect we had for food. We celebrated everything we ate."

While Gennaro's father and grandfather lived for a long time, it was his grandmother who was truly impressive, reaching the age of 101. He believes that the importance she placed on tasty food helped her live as long and healthily as she did.

"Flavour is key for good health," he says. When you eat well and really enjoy your food you're left feeling properly satisfied and therefore not likely to overeat, says Gennaro. "Good flavour makes your body happy, and when your body is happy it's also healthy."

Our conversation is suddenly interrupted by a knock at the door. It's his friend Pasqualino, who's after a snack. "He's always visiting and he's very picky," says Gennaro, jumping up from his seat. Pasqualino, it turns out, is a rather large squirrel waiting on his hind legs outside the glass door to the kitchen. Inviting him in, Gennaro hands Pasqualino a walnut in its shell, which the furry creature clasps in his paws, inspects diligently for a few moments – "quality control", explains Gennaro – before scampering off and promptly being replaced by another. "This is his friend, Francescelo," Gennaro tells me. "They just love these fresh walnuts. I think about what they're going to like."

I think we need to take feeding ourselves as seriously as Gennaro takes feeding his squirrels.

Never eat out of obligation

Giovanna Trimarchi from Molochio, whom we met in Part 3, told me that not once in her 93 years has she eaten anything because she felt that she should; something she considered dull but "good for her". Instead, she's spent a lifetime putting flavour first – whatever she makes, she makes it delicious.

When flavour is at the forefront of decision-making, you never have to eat out of obligation. Life is too short to eat things you don't enjoy and there is also no need. If you don't like cabbage, don't eat cabbage. Experiment with ingredients and ways of cooking until you find the recipes that really delight you and that you actively look forward to.

The good news is that, from the broad food groups discussed in this book that we know are good for our health, there are literally endless options for dinner. In modern times "healthy" food has become associated with boring or tasteless food. This is completely untrue. The foods of Italy or Japan are among the world's most revered for their flavour and yet both cuisines are also very good for you. Middle Eastern cooking, packed with delicious herbs, spices and legumes, is bursting with goodness. Healthy food is flavoursome food.

The bottom line is, make all your meals something you really want to eat.

2. Don't go for convenience

A simple strategy for improving your health is to cook your own meals from real, honest ingredients, like the blue-zoners do. That way you know exactly what's in your food and can make it in exactly the way you like. You don't have to hand over the decision of what ingredients to put in your body to big food companies who are not, as of yet, incentivised to think about your health.

I sometimes wonder what future generations will think of our contemporary diet. Maybe in the future we will be more reliant than ever on UPFs. But somehow, I think not. Because industrially produced "food" is doing us harm and we are beginning to realise this.

Cooking real food is an act of self-care and taking pride in what you eat is valuing yourself.

Seek out and celebrate good produce; get in touch with where your food has come from; see the simple wonder in basic things like beans or old bread; really taste your food. Marvel at fresh fish, warm ricotta, soothing fennel, shiny red tomatoes and buttery walnuts. Make food that really makes your heart sing, your brain happy and your stomach satisfied. This is the true meaning of eating healthily and you won't find it in a packet.

What about the cost?

The cost of real, nutritious food is an enormous, glaring issue in the UK. One that governments are repeatedly failing to address.

At the moment, we are living in a society where all sorts

of normal, staple, necessary foods are simply unaffordable to many people, which is a preposterous, shameful situation to find ourselves in. And shortsighted. Whatever the government would spend in implementing a subsidy would be more than covered by the corresponding reduction in the enormous cost of treating obesity and other chronic illnesses that are caused by poor nutrition.

As we heard from Italy's blue-zoners, their traditional diet was based on plants, which were cheap and abundant, while meat and sweet foods were pricey and less accessible. In the modern world, in the UK, this hierarchy has been flipped on its head. Ultra-processed, sweetened products and poor-quality meat are among the cheapest foods available, whereas fresh vegetables and fruit are now beyond the means of many people.

It can sometimes be hard to get to grips with this situation. Just know that you don't need to be buying expensive kale or avocados to improve your diet. Any vegetables, legumes and nuts will do, so buy what you can afford – frozen peas and spinach are always in my freezer, and my cupboard is never without cheap and nutritious tins of beans.

What if you just love convenience?

If it's a question of loving the convenience and speed of modern-day food-like products, remember that it's a false economy. You might save time in the short term, but you could be lining up health problems in the long term. Not so convenient.

There are meals you can make from scratch that are

almost instant, as well as satisfying and nutritious.

My go-tos for when I have little time are frittatas of any kind (cheese, peas, courgettes, herbs) or salads with leaves from a bag, jarred vegetables like artichokes and peppers, any kind of nuts or seeds, chickpeas, a little cheese or a boiled egg and a simple dressing of olive oil and vinegar. A stir-fry of vegetables with noodles and tofu is also super-quick. Real fast food will fill you up and make you happier than any ready-meal ever can.

Unfortunately, it's not so easy when you're out and about. Nearly all of our ready-to-eat food from high-street chains is ultra-processed and very bad value for money. The way I got around this when working from an office was to bring in my leftovers from dinner the night before or something that I could quickly assemble in the morning. This worked out cheaper, more filling, more varied and more nutritious than any of the options available to buy near the office.

Prioritise eating well just as you'd prioritise the gym or washing your hair

Of course, preparing food for yourself takes time – it won't just magically appear before you. But prioritising proper nourishment, the way you might prioritise going to the gym or other things you do for health, such as cleaning your teeth, will improve your wellbeing, help you maintain a healthy weight and increase the likelihood that you'll make it into old age like a blue-zoner. For an extra 15 minutes in the kitchen, this is worth your while. Try and embrace slower cooking too. There is a lot of fun to be had there.

Another thing I want to tell you is that absolutely anyone

can cook. It's not a skill reserved for only a talented few; it's a universal ability that anyone with a chopping board, a knife and a pan can access. You don't have to make things up; pick a clearly written recipe with a few simple steps and an outcome you like the sound of. If it doesn't go to plan, it's probably that the recipe is badly written – not your lack of ability. Don't become despondent; just try a different recipe. The more times you make something you like, the more confident you'll become in your skills and the more creative your cooking will get. After a while, you'll be able to create simple, tasty dishes on a whim from bits and bobs in your fridge and cupboards – an old courgette, some pasta and some cheese can result in a stunning dish worthy of the Amalfi coast.

3. Eat seasonally

Cooking seasonally is another key way to eat yourself happy. Since people in the blue zones tend to grow their own food, or buy it from someone else who has grown it, everything they eat (bar preserves) is seasonal.

This is beneficial for a number of reasons. First, fresher fruit and vegetables, picked close to harvest, taste really good. Secondly, they contain more nutrients. The longer fruit and veg are stored or transported, the more their nutrients decline. Thirdly, it's a great way to introduce natural variation into your diet, and so improve your gut diversity. You will also appreciate ingredients more when they're not available to you all year round.

Think about how good mince pies taste because we only have them once a year – the same thing is true of fruits and vegetables. You can't beat a crisp, tart autumn apple, comforting chestnuts and colourful squash in deepest, darkest winter; the first of the sweet and delicate asparagus in May; and bright, juicy blackberries in summer. You learn to savour them when they're not consumed all the time in a boring monotony; and when you do eat them, they'll be at the peak of their flavour.

Another perk of eating seasonally is that it can be very economical. Fruit and veg that's in season will tend to be cheaper, especially at food markets where sellers do deals on produce they have a lot of. In big cities, like London, there are plenty of good markets; most towns have one or two as well. If you live in a rural area, then farm shops are a great place to get quality British produce. There are also a number of online retailers that will deliver seasonal fruit and veg to your door.

If you don't know what's in season at a particular time of the year, you're not alone. Our supermarket shelves look pretty much the same all year round. If you want to buy tomatoes or strawberries in winter, you very easily can. If you want to eat a pear in June, that's absolutely fine! *Be our guest*, say the supermarkets, *it's only travelled 9,000 miles to get here.*

That's not to say I'm entirely against modernity – I don't think you should live your life without ever eating a banana or a mango, for example, that do not grow here. But for maximum taste – which is crucial for a happy diet – and as a nourishing way to mark the beauty of nature and its rhythms, eating seasonally when possible makes a lot of sense.

One of the nicest things about eating this way is that

when ingredients are in season, they don't need a lot of work to make them shine. This, really, is the unspectacular secret behind Italian cooking: they just pick ingredients that are at their best and let those ingredients speak for themselves. A great Italian chef and friend of mine, Francesco Mazzei, originally from Calabria but now living in London, remembers the wonderful cooking of his nonna.

"If you have the best tomato, the best onion and the best cucumber, all you need is extra-virgin olive oil – you don't even need salt. We tend to overdress things now and I think that's because, by not following the seasons, our food is lacking in taste." The culture of seeking out the best aubergine or the ripest, most beautiful fig is the uncomplicated power of Italian cuisine, says Francesco.

"One time when she was in her nineties, I bought Nonna some fennel in summer – she looked at it like a monster. 'Where did you get this from?' she asked me. 'America? ... No, no, no, it's not good'."

We might not have the same produce as either Italy or Costa Rica in the UK, but we have a whole host of our own wonderful fruit and vegetables that grow fantastically here and taste incredible.

You can find helpful lists online of what's in season when.

4. Eat together

It's not always possible to eat together, but when the opportunity presents itself, grab it. Whether it's a sandwich with a colleague on a bench, a plate of spaghetti with your partner at your kitchen table or a massive feast with your mates down at the local curry house, it will make you feel good.

Sharing a meal with somebody, as we learnt earlier, is not only something that brings happiness in the short term; it facilitates bonding, making you feel less lonely and more content in the long term. It also makes the whole act of eating more conscious and deliberate, minimising the likelihood that you'll sit there and mindlessly overeat.

In the blue zones, the highly communal way of eating is perhaps as great a contributor to their health as their nutritious diet. Eating together – and making mealtimes important – offers everybody at the table a specific time to socialise, connect and relax. It may be the only time you get in your day to really talk to your loved ones without any distractions.

Sitting down to dinner with my friends or family, or a combination of the two, is one of my favourite things to do, especially when the food is in the middle and everyone can help themselves. There is something about passing plates to one another, sharing the experience of eating the same food and showing gratitude en masse to whoever made it that is incredibly enriching.

Sharing food sparks conversation, laughter and love. My favourite memories of my nonna and grandad are around the table.

In a world where our attention is often divided and many of us feel like we're constantly rushing from place to place, mealtimes are a natural pause in the day for enjoyment and connection. And couldn't we all do with more of that?

5. Above all, don't "diet"

What do we associate with the word "diet" in the West? Normally: restriction, discipline, a wrestle with willpower, moral superiority, shame, short-term effects followed by long-term "failure", meals that leave us feeling, in one way or another, unsatisfied…

But the word diet was never meant to convey these things. It comes from the Greek *diaita*, which means "a way of life" and this is the best way to think about what and how you eat. *Diaita* is crucial to understanding the effectiveness of the blue-zone diet.

Most modern diets force you to live in the extremes, in the granular; they advocate peculiar or hard-to-live-with measures that are apparently perfectly doable if only you have the willpower to stick with the programme.

People whose message is "eat like me, look like me" are lying to you. We are all individuals with different bodies and requirements. Blunt and intense practices, such as cutting out all carbohydrates, might work for them but not for you.

Instead, trust your own instincts. For example, I like to eat my main meal in the middle of the day and in general don't have any appetite before about 10 or 11am. My friend jokes that I'm a snake, preferring a feast and long digestion period to more frequent, smaller meals. She, on the other hand, can always eat breakfast, regardless of how early it is. She eats a smaller lunch than me and never skips dinner. We are exactly the same height and weight.

Moreover, even if going on an extreme diet can "work" in the short term, is that really how you want to live your life? There is such a thing in psychology as "arrival fallacy". It is the false notion that once we achieve our goals we will be rewarded with everlasting happiness. Sadly, the "reward" at the end of a diet is that you have to maintain that diet *for ever*. Do you want to maintain a strict diet *for ever*? Do you never want to eat foods you really enjoy again? Is it even possible? We know from the science that the answer is a resounding no.

A study from UCLA in 2007 found that two-thirds of dieters regained more weight than they lost on their diet once they'd stopped it.[146] In fact, dieting is a consistent and robust predictor of weight gain, with research suggesting that the more attempts you make to lose weight, the more likely you are to gain it in the future.[147]

Do not be fooled by people promising miraculous results via restrictive methods that will only set you up for a fraught relationship with food. Intense regimes might work for some people but only for so long and will only propel you into a cycle of perceived success and failure. This is no way to look at food or to live your life. You're better off changing and enhancing the way you eat in general than doing something extreme and niche in the short term.

Good health is about the way you eat and the way you live your life *most of the time*, which means there's no need for obsession or guilt *ever*. It's a boring cliché, but I fully subscribe to the philosophy of everything in moderation, including moderation. Even though I know it's not good for me (in one sense), sometimes I want to go to the pub with my friends and drink multiple pints of beer. I'm not going to feel bad about that. True wellbeing lies in ease, not strict rules.

In essence, think about your *diaita*, not a short-lived fix.

Lose weight without obsessing over it

There's nothing wrong with wanting to lose weight. And, if this is your goal, eating in a way that constantly prioritises real flavour and dismisses food neuroticism will help you more than any diet you've ever done. To reiterate, this means making all food really tasty, whether it's broccoli or a slice of Victoria sponge.

A focus on eating real food, with the incorporation of lots of plants, will make you feel more satisfied and nourished than a diet of UPFs, which means there's much less chance you'll overeat – it's hard to consume too many beans but it's easy to eat too many Doritos. And remember: plants doesn't just mean vegetables but legumes, nuts, spices, herbs, fruit and grains too.

By eating nutrient-dense meals made with real, tasty ingredients, you'll naturally know when to stop eating. You won't have to obsess about your diet. You won't have to even think about it.

The happiest diet in the world

An easy, loving, celebratory relationship with food is what makes the diets of the world's longevity hotspots so successful. This, in summary, is their *diaita*:

🌶 Their food is plant-rich, meaning they eat everything from leafy greens and potatoes to walnuts and mushrooms; from daikon and chickpeas to rosemary and radishes; from oranges and figs to ginger and black pepper. Eating with the seasons brings natural variety and diversity.

🍂 They cook their meals themselves and do not eat industrially prepared food. Ultra-processed snacks like biscuits or crisps were unheard of until recently and did not feature in the diets of the now elderly.

🍂 Meat is an occasional treat. The consumption of fish, though greater than meat, is still moderate.

🍂 Dairy is either very fresh or fermented into yoghurt and cheese.

🍂 Legumes play a prominent role in the diet, with many recipes based around them. In some communities they are eaten every day.

🍂 Nuts of all sorts are also important and eaten frequently.

🍂 Desserts, at least in the past, had to be homemade, but still today are only eaten occasionally.

🍂 Bread, also homemade, is baked using the traditional sourdough method, resulting in a very different product from the ultra-processed, very sweet loaves in our supermarkets in the West.

🍂 Small glasses of red wine (just one or two) are enjoyed frequently, but normally with food and in company.

🌶 Extra-virgin olive oil is the preferred oil for both cooking and eating and is consumed in abundance.

🌶 Meals are normally eaten communally and are recognised as an important time to socialise.

🌶 Food is celebrated, not demonised or associated with guilt.

🌶 Whether intentional, like the Japanese philosophy of getting up from the table 80 per cent full, or circumstantial, as caused by the food shortages during the war in Molochio, there is an ingrained understanding of the value of occasional abstinence.

There's nothing exceptional or extreme about blue-zone eating. It's not mind-blowing or "sexy" or complicated and you don't need a degree in nutrition to understand it. If anything, it offers a message based on an instinctive wisdom, a wisdom that in recent decades has got lost under so much confusing and conflicting advice: eat plenty of plants, cook your own food, save sugary treats for occasions and generally don't overindulge.

What is special about blue-zone eating is that it's never a chore. It's not "healthy" eating; it's just delicious food achieved through care and love. Making food for somebody is one of life's great pleasures, because it communicates to them their importance to you; the same goes for what you make for yourself. Cooking simple meals is one of the most important things you can do for yourself in terms of your health, your happiness and the way you age, and, once learnt, will be an easy habit you have for life, opening the door to a whole new world of flavour and experiences.

By tapping into ancient food wisdom, which continues to be validated by ever-growing food science, and reconnecting with true nourishment, you can transform your life one plate at a time and maybe even live to 100.

I have always believed in the wisdom of grandmothers, and it turns out they were on to something. So, as mine would have said: "*Mangia, mangia.*"

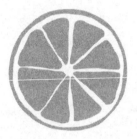

RECIPES

All these recipes are about enjoyment first and health second, which allow you to access good nutrition without even thinking about it – like they do in the blue zones. There are plenty of plants, legumes, nuts and olive oil, of course, but nothing is excluded because nothing needs to be. That's why you'll find meat dishes and delicious desserts too.

SPRING

Broad beans with ricotta on sourdough

What a way to upgrade your toast. I adore this combo of creamy, citrusy ricotta and mild, nutty, sweet broad beans (a hero legume).

Prep time: 10 minutes
Serves 2

2 slices of sourdough bread, toasted
1 garlic clove, peeled
100g ricotta cheese
zest of ½ lemon
120g broad beans, boiled for 3–4 minutes if fresh, 5–6 minutes if frozen, and peeled
2 tsp olive oil
½ tsp chilli flakes (optional)
salt and pepper

1. Rub the garlic clove all over one side of the toasted sourdough. Save what's left of the garlic for another dish – you won't need it all.
2. Mix the ricotta with the lemon zest and season with salt and pepper. Spread over the toast, top with the broad beans and a drizzle of olive oil. Finish with the chilli flakes, if using, and a pinch of salt and pepper.

Watercress and basil soup with toasted walnuts

Bright, fresh, fragrant and comes together in 20 minutes. The toasted walnuts complete it with their buttery warmth.

Prep time: 10 minutes
Cook time: 20 minutes
Serves 4

1 medium onion, peeled and finely chopped
2 celery sticks, finely chopped
1 small potato, peeled and cut into 1cm cubes
1 garlic clove, peeled and roughly chopped
2 tbsp olive oil
900ml vegetable or chicken stock
240g watercress
4 sprigs of basil (use leaves and stalks)
juice of ½ lemon
60g walnuts, toasted in a dry frying pan and roughly chopped
salt and pepper

1. Place the onion, celery, potato and olive oil in a medium saucepan over a low heat. Cover with a lid and sweat for 10 minutes, removing the lid to stir from time to time. Add the garlic and cook for 1 minute more.
2. Pour in the stock, increase the heat slightly to bring it to a simmer. Cover and cook for 8 minutes.
3. Add the watercress and cook for a scant minute. Remove from the heat, add the basil and blitz with a stick blender until smooth. Stir in the lemon juice, season and serve topped with toasted walnuts. A drizzle of olive oil also makes a nice addition.

Broccoli and anchovy pasta

These two ingredients really are the best of friends – the deep umami flavour of the anchovies cutting through the subtle bitterness of broccoli. Remember to finish it with some beautiful extra virgin olive oil.

Prep time: 10 minutes
Cook time: 10 minutes
Serves 2

150g orecchiette pasta
1 head of broccoli, cut into small florets
5 tbsp olive oil
3 garlic cloves, peeled
6 anchovies from a jar
1 red chilli
juice of ½ lemon
salt and pepper

1. Cook the pasta in a saucepan of generously salted water for 8 minutes or until al dente.
2. While the pasta is cooking, finely chop the garlic, anchovies and chilli and mix them together to form a rough paste.
3. Two minutes before the pasta is ready, add the broccoli to the saucepan. Drain and reserve 2 tablespoons of the cooking water.
4. Place a large frying pan on a medium heat and sauté the paste in the olive oil for 1½ minutes. Add the pasta and broccoli, along with the reserved pasta water, mix everything together and keep on the heat for 1 minute longer. Season to taste (bearing in mind the anchovies are salty), stir in the lemon juice and serve.

Radicchio, orange and feta salad with toasted walnuts

This gorgeous salad is bitter, sweet, bright, salty and tangy all at the same time, with added crunch from the walnuts. It also works well with pecans or hazelnuts.

Prep time: 15 minutes
Serves 2

For the dressing:
juice of ½ orange
3 tbsp olive oil
1 tbsp white wine vinegar
1 tsp honey
2 tsp Dijon mustard
salt and pepper

For the salad:
2 medium oranges, peeled
30g walnuts
1 small radicchio, finely shredded
5 radishes, finely sliced
100g feta cheese

1. Place all the ingredients for the dressing in a bowl and whisk until emulsified. Season with salt and pepper.
2. Peel the oranges and slice each one into ½cm rounds. Cut each round into four.
3. Toast the walnuts in a dry frying pan until golden and fragrant, then roughly chop.
4. Place all the salad ingredients in a serving dish, then toss them in the dressing and season with a pinch of salt and pepper before serving.

Cabbage and pecorino gratin

This gratin is a total treat – rich, unctuous caramelised cabbage with a deliciously crunchy topping.

Prep time: 10 minutes
Cook time: 40 minutes
Serves 4

1 onion, peeled and finely sliced
3 sprigs of thyme, leaves picked
3 tbsp olive oil
1 medium savoy cabbage, sliced into 8 wedges
170g pecorino, finely grated
3 tbsp crème fraîche
1 tbsp Dijon mustard

For the topping:
50g panko breadcrumbs
2 tbsp olive oil
3 sprigs of thyme, leaves picked
salt and pepper

1. Preheat the oven to 200°C/180°C fan/gas mark 6. Place the onion, thyme and 2 tablespoons of olive oil in a large shallow casserole dish (the one I used was 30cm in diameter) and sauté on a medium heat for 7 minutes, or until the onions are softened and turning golden.
2. Arrange the cabbage wedges in a single layer on top of the onions and add 100–150ml water. Cover with a lid and sweat for 10 minutes.
3. Mix the grated pecorino, crème fraîche and Dijon mustard together with a pinch of salt and pepper. Add

2–3 tablespoons of water to loosen the mixture so it resembles a bechamel sauce.

4. Remove the lid and pour the sauce over the cabbage, covering as much of it as possible. Transfer to the oven, uncovered, for 12 minutes.

5. To make the topping, mix the breadcrumbs with the olive oil, thyme and a pinch of salt and pepper, ensuring that they are thoroughly coated. Scatter over the gratin and return to the oven for 8–10 minutes longer, or until the breadcrumbs are golden and crisp and the edges of the gratin are beginning to caramelise.

Asparagus, tarragon and Parmesan risotto

Stirring risotto offers a brilliant opportunity to pause and wind down. I love watching the rice transform from hard and uncooked to plump and perfectly done, as it soaks up all the delicious liquid. This is a dish that will make everyone very happy.

Prep time: 10 minutes
Cook time: 45 minutes
Serves 4

1.3 litres chicken or vegetable stock
5 tbsp olive oil
1 onion, peeled and finely diced
2 garlic cloves, peeled and finely chopped
250g arborio rice
150ml white wine
250g asparagus, finely sliced into little rounds
4 sprigs of tarragon, finely chopped
50g Parmesan, finely grated
½ lemon, to serve

1. Put the stock into a large saucepan over a medium heat and bring to a very gentle simmer. Heat 3 tablespoons of olive oil in a large frying pan over a low heat and fry the onion for 7–8 minutes, stirring occasionally, until starting to turn golden. Add the garlic and cook for 1–2 minutes more.
2. Pour in the rice- stir until it is well coated and cook, constantly stirring, for 3–4 minutes until the outside of the grains become translucent.
3. Add the wine and stir until it has been absorbed. Now

add a generous ladleful of stock and stir again until absorbed. Continue this process until you have about 2 ladlefuls of liquid left. It takes about 20–25 minutes.

4. Add the asparagus and tarragon, stir to combine and add half the remaining stock. When absorbed, pour in what is left. When the stock has been used, the rice should be soft with a little bit of bite.

5. Stir in the Parmesan, remaining olive oil and season to taste. Allow the risotto to rest for 4–5 minutes before serving with a squeeze of lemon juice and some extra olive oil if desired.

Slow-cooked leg of lamb with crispy potatoes

My grandad's favourite garlic and rosemary studded lamb! Cooked this way, the lamb becomes super soft, tender and sweet and is amazing with the garlicky, olive-oily cubed potatoes. Serve with whatever veg you fancy.

Prep time: 20 minutes
Cook time: 6 hours
Serves 6

1 bulb of garlic
1.3kg leg of lamb
6 sprigs of rosemary
300ml chicken stock
1kg potatoes, cut into 1cm cubes
3 sprigs of thyme, leaves picked
7 tbsp olive oil

1. Preheat the oven to 150'C/130'C fan/gas 2. Separate the garlic cloves from the bulb and peel each one. Set aside 2 cloves for the potatoes and slice 4 of them in half.
2. Use a sharp knife to make deep incisions all over the lamb and stuff each one with the sliced garlic. Cut 3 sprigs of rosemary into 2cm-long pieces and stuff these into the incisions with the garlic.
3. Place the lamb in a medium roasting tin. Pour in the stock and add any remaining garlic cloves and rosemary. Drizzle 4 tablespoons of olive oil over the lamb, season it with salt and freshly ground pepper and cover tightly with foil. Transfer to the oven for 6 hours.
4. Two hours before the lamb is ready, finely chop the 2 reserved garlic cloves and add to a bowl with 3 table-

spoons of olive oil and the thyme leaves. Season generously with salt and pepper.

5. Toss the potatoes in the oil mixture and lay them in a single layer on a large baking tray. Roast in the same oven for 1 hour 45 minutes, turning a few times throughout cooking, to make sure they cook and crisp evenly.

6. When the lamb is ready, transfer it from the tray to a board, cover with foil and allow it to rest for 10–15 minutes. Place the roasting dish on a medium heat and deglaze the pan with the remaining chicken stock for a couple of minutes. Pass through a sieve and season. Serve alongside the lamb and potatoes.

Tip
The potatoes can be cooked any time within the 6-hour window of cooking the lamb, and reheated before serving.)

Spring vegetable minestrone

Longevity in a bowl. This soup tastes phenomenal.

Prep time: 15 minutes
Cook time: 1hr 10 minutes
Serves 6

3 tbsp olive oil
1 leek, quartered lengthways and finely sliced
2 carrots, peeled and finely diced
2 celery sticks, finely diced
3 garlic cloves, peeled and finely chopped
2 tbsp tomato purée
1 400g tin chopped tomatoes
1 400g tin cannellini beans
1 courgette, quartered lengthways and diced
250g asparagus, cut into 1cm pieces
150g frozen broad beans
30g bunch of basil, finely shredded
1.3 litres chicken or vegetable stock
100g pasta (small macaroni or similar)
15–20g Parmesan, for serving

1. Heat the olive oil in a large saucepan over a medium heat and add the leek, carrots and celery. Season with a pinch of salt and sauté for 10–12 minutes, stirring occasionally. Add the garlic and cook for 1 minute more.
2. Make a space in the centre of the pan and cook the tomato purée for a few minutes, before mixing it in. Tip in the tomatoes, season again and simmer for about 15 minutes, or until the sauce is beginning to thicken.
3. Add the cannellini beans, courgette, asparagus, broad beans, basil and stock. Stir everything together, cover with

a lid and simmer for 25 minutes.
4. Remove the lid, add the pasta and cook for about 12 minutes, or until al dente. Season to taste, and serve with some Parmesan a squeeze of lemon and a drizzle of olive oil.

Warm potato salad with capers, dill and lemon

I love baby new potatoes with just butter and salt but here, in this tangy, salty, herby dressing they taste divine. Chopped anchovies make a great addition.

Prep time: 10 minutes
Cook time: 20 minutes
Serves 4 (as a side)

650g baby new potatoes
60g rocket, finely chopped
15g dill, roughly chopped
40g capers, drained
zest of 1 lemon and juice of half
1 tsp red wine vinegar
4 tbsp olive oil
salt and pepper

1. Place the baby potatoes in a medium saucepan with a generous pinch of salt, cover with water, bring to the boil and simmer for 15–20 minutes, or until tender.
2. Meanwhile, mix together the rest of the ingredients in a serving bowl. When the potatoes are ready, drain them and allow them to steam dry for a few minutes, then toss them in the dressing. Serve while still warm.

Chickpeas with clams, garlic and parsley

This is such a delicious recipe and really easy to make – don't be put off by the clam prep, it's more straightforward than you think. The combination of salty clams, sweet, nutty chickpeas and the comforting aroma of wine, lemon and parsley will transport you to the sunshine of a blue zone.

Prep time: 10 minutes
Cook time: 15 minutes
Serves 2

800g clams
90ml (6 tbsp) olive oil
1 onion, peeled and finely chopped
5 garlic cloves, peeled and finely chopped
120ml white wine
1 400g tin chickpeas, drained and rinsed
20g parsley, finely chopped
salt and pepper
lemon wedges to serve

1. First, sort through the clams. Clean them and discard any which are open and which don't close immediately when tapped on the countertop.
2. Place a large, wide casserole dish on a medium heat and sauté the onion in the olive oil for 10 minutes. Add the garlic and cook for 1 minute more.
3. Increase the heat to high, add the white wine, clams and chickpeas and give the pan a vigorous shake to mix everything together. Cover with a tight-fitting lid and cook for 3–4 minutes, or until all the clam shells have

popped open, shaking the pan from time to time to help things along.

4. Remove from the heat, season with a generous pinch of salt and pepper, and add the parsley. Mix one more time and serve immediately with some lemon wedges on the side. Remember not to eat any clams that have not opened. Serve with crusty bread to mop up the delicious juices.

SUMMER

Artichokes with parsley and hazelnuts

Artichokes have such an exquisite and unique flavour. They are also an excellent prebiotic – food for your gut microbes – and a rich source of polyphenols. They can be hard to prep so this recipe, using jarred ones, makes things super easy.

Prep time: 8 minutes
Serves 2

50g hazelnuts
20g parsley, finely chopped
4 tbsp olive oil
1½ tbsp red wine vinegar
1 tsp Dijon mustard
salt and pepper
2 jars of artichokes in oil, drained

1. Toast the hazelnuts in a dry frying pan for a couple of minutes, until golden all over. When ready, roughly chop and transfer to a bowl.
2. Add the parsley, olive oil, red wine vinegar, Dijon mustard and a generous pinch of salt and pepper. Mix to combine.
3. Arrange the artichokes in a serving dish and spoon the dressing all over.

Fish soup

The beauty of this soup is that it works with a wide range of fish or shellfish – just choose what you fancy or what's in season. Not everyone will have easy access to mussels, for example, in which case stick to fish – simply increase the quantity you use to 550g in total. Prawns also make a nice addition.

Prep time: 5 minutes
Cook time: 35 minutes
Serves 4

3 garlic cloves, peeled and sliced
3 sprigs of thyme, leaves picked
2 tbsp olive oil
400g tin chopped tomatoes
2 tbsp capers plus 1 tbsp their pickling juice
100ml white wine
400g tin haricot beans, drained and rinsed
800ml fish stock
450g mix of fish, such as cod, salmon and monkfish, skin removed and cut into 2cm chunks
400g mussels, scrubbed and beards removed
salt and pepper
2 tbsp dill or parsley, roughly chopped (optional)

1. In a large saucepan, sauté the garlic and thyme with the olive oil for 1–2 minutes or until fragrant. Add the chopped tomatoes, capers and their juice and white wine, plus a pinch of salt, and simmer for 10–15 minutes.
2. Pour in the haricot beans and stock and continue to cook for a further 10 minutes.
3. Carefully lower the fish and mussels into the sauce,

cover with a lid and cook for 8–10 minutes, or until the mussel shells have opened (discard any that don't). Scatter over the chopped dill or parsley, and finish with a drizzle of olive oil.

Mozzarella with anchovies, lemon and parsley

Zesty, creamy, salty... this salad has it all.

Prep time: 10 minutes
Serves 2

5 anchovies, roughly chopped
7–8 sprigs of parsley, leaves picked and finely chopped
zest and juice of 1 lemon
4 tbsp olive oil
3 medium-ripe plum tomatoes, each sliced into ½cm rounds
1 ball of mozzarella
salt

1. Mix the anchovies, parsley, lemon zest and half the lemon juice in a bowl with 2 tablespoons of olive oil.
2. Layer the tomatoes in a serving dish and season with a pinch of salt. Drizzle the remaining olive oil and lemon juice all over.
3. Tear the mozzarella open and lay it on top of the tomatoes. Spoon the anchovy relish on top and serve with crusty bread.

Creamed chard on toast

This recipe really celebrates the wonder of chard – the dark leafy green with a subtle, bitter flavour. It's among the most nutrient-dense foods in the world, and is packed with fibre. I like to serve this recipe as an alternative to traditional bruschetta.

Prep time: 5 minutes
Cook time: 12 minutes
Serves 2

1 banana shallot, peeled and finely chopped
2 tbsp olive oil
200g chard, leaves and stalks finely shredded
¼ nutmeg, finely grated
1 tbsp crème fraîche
2 slices sourdough, toasted
1 garlic clove, peeled
Salt and pepper

1. Place a large frying pan (one with a lid) on a medium heat with the olive oil and sauté the shallot for 5–6 minutes, until softened.
2. Add the chard stalks and sauté these for 3–4 minutes. Then stir in the shredded chard leaves, cover with a lid and sweat for 4 minutes. Lift the lid to stir halfway through.
3. Remove from the heat and add the nutmeg and crème fraîche. Stir to combine and season with salt and pepper.
4. Rub each slice of toast lightly with garlic and serve topped with the creamed chard, and an extra drizzle of olive oil.

Peas with mustard and dill

So simple, so tasty. A great way to celebrate a very healthy legume. This dish is lovely served with fish.

Prep time: 5 minutes
Cook time: 5 minutes
Serves 2 as a main, 4 as a side

3 tbsp olive oil
1 tbsp mustard seeds
500g peas, podded if fresh, defrosted if frozen
1 tbsp Dijon mustard
10g dill, finely chopped
salt and pepper
juice of ½ lemon

1. Heat the olive oil in a medium casserole dish with a tight-fitting lid and add the mustard seeds. Cook for about 30 seconds or until they start to pop.
2. Add the peas, mustard and dill and mix together well. Pour in 2 tablespoons of water, reduce the heat to low and cover with a lid. Braise for 4 minutes, if using frozen peas (6 minutes if using fresh from the pod).
3. Season with salt and pepper, stir in the lemon juice and serve.

Green beans in tomato sauce

This is a classic southern Italian recipe that celebrates the humble green bean. Great as part of a big spread.

Prep time: 5 minutes
Cook time: 1hr 10 minutes
Serves 2 as a main, 4 as a side

1 onion, finely chopped
4 tbsp olive oil
2 garlic cloves, peeled and roughly chopped
400g tin chopped tomatoes
2 sprigs of thyme, leaves picked
250g green beans, trimmed
4 sprigs of basil (use leaves and stalks)
1 tsp red wine vinegar
salt and pepper
15–20g pecorino (or Parmesan)

1. Place the onion in a pan with 2 tablespoons of the olive oil and a pinch of salt. Sauté for 10 minutes, until soft. Add the garlic and cook for 1 minute more.
2. Stir in the chopped tomatoes, thyme and 100ml water. Season, cover with a lid and simmer for 50 minutes or until the flavours are concentrated and the sauce has reduced slightly.
3. In a separate pan, parboil the beans for 3–4 minutes, then add them with the basil and red wine vinegar to the pan with the tomato sauce, tossing everything lightly to coat. Cook on a medium heat for 8–10 minutes, or until the green beans are tender.
4. Serve drizzled with the remaining olive oil, shavings of pecorino and some black pepper.

Aubergine parmigiana

I think this is the ultimate vegetarian dish. I love the crispy, caramelised bits of aubergine you get round the edges along with the umami of the tomato sauce and the creaminess of the melted mozzarella. Note that aubergines act like sponges and absorb the olive oil quickly so liberal amounts are required.

Prep time: 15 minutes
Cook time: 1hr 45 minutes
Serves 6

4 medium aubergines, sliced into ½cm rounds
8–9 tbsp olive oil
1 onion, peeled and finely chopped
2 garlic cloves, peeled and finely chopped
2 400g tins chopped tomatoes
40g basil
2 balls of mozzarella
40g Parmesan
salt and pepper

1. Lay the aubergine slices in a tray or flat dish, scatter generously with sea salt and set aside while you make the tomato sauce.
2. Heat 2 tablespoons of olive oil in a medium saucepan. Sauté the onion with a pinch of salt over a low heat for 8 minutes, or until softened. Add the garlic and cook for 1 minute more.
3. Stir in the tomatoes and 200ml water, along with half of the basil and another pinch of salt. Cover with a lid and simmer for 30 minutes, stirring occasionally.
4. Pour 2 tablespoons of olive oil into a large frying pan

and turn the heat to high. When hot, add a layer of aubergines and fry on both sides until golden brown. Continue to cook the slices in batches, adding a tablespoon of oil each time, and setting them aside on layers of kitchen paper after removing them from the pan.

5. Preheat the oven to 200°C/180°C fan/gas mark 6. To assemble the parmigiana, start with a layer of aubergines in the base of a deep-sided baking dish (approx. 20 x 20cm). Spoon some tomato sauce over, followed by some basil leaves, torn mozzarella and grated Parmesan. Repeat this process three more times, finishing with tomato sauce and cheese on top.

6. Drizzle with a little extra olive oil, then transfer to the oven and bake for 30 minutes, or until golden, crispy and bubbling. Serve with a lightly dressed rocket salad.

Sardines with tomatoes, capers, lemon and basil

Sardines are deliciously good for you, full of anti-inflammatory, cardioprotective omega-3 fatty acid. But they're not always easy to buy fresh, so we've made sure this recipe works well with tinned (which, because of the soft bones, are an even better source of calcium). If you do go for fresh, they just need to be fried for a few minutes on each side until crispy and browned.

Prep time: 15 minutes
Serves 2

350g cherry tomatoes, quartered
20g rocket, very finely chopped
20g basil, finely shredded
1½ tbsp capers
juice of 1 lemon
½ tsp chilli flakes (optional)
3 tbsp olive oil
salt and pepper
140g tin of sardines (best quality you can afford)

1. Place the tomatoes, rocket and basil in a large bowl.
2. Roughly chop the capers and mix with the lemon juice, chilli flakes, olive oil and some seasoning. Pour over the tomatoes and toss to coat.
3. Divide the mixture between two dishes and top each with two sardines. Serve immediately.

Tip
Turn the salad into a panzanella by adding chunks of stale sourdough or other bread to soak up the juices. You will need an extra glug of olive oil.

Cannellini beans with chicken, sage and tomatoes

Tender, succulent meat with crispy skin and soft, flavoursome beans infused with the wonderful flavour of sage. Nourishing through and through.

Prep time: 10 minutes
Cook time: 2hrs 45 minutes
Serves 2

90ml olive oil
2 chicken legs
3 shallots, finely chopped
1 medium leek, finely sliced
4 cloves garlic, finely sliced
8 plum tomatoes (700g roughly), each one roughly cut into 8 chunks
400g tin cannellini beans, drained and rinsed
110ml chicken stock
25g sage, leaves picked
1 tbsp capers
½ lemon, sliced in 4 and pips removed
salt and pepper

1. Preheat the oven to 140°C/120°C fan/gas mark 1. Place a large casserole dish on a medium heat with 3 tablespoons of olive oil. Salt the chicken legs and fry them until they are golden all over – roughly 10 minutes – then set aside.
2. Add the shallots, leek and garlic to the pan and sauté for 8–10 minutes, or until fragrant and beginning to soften.
3. Add the remaining ingredients, along with a generous

pinch of salt and pepper. Stir well and bring to the boil. Place the chicken legs on top of the mixture and press down until they are almost fully submerged in the sauce, leaving the skin exposed.

4. Transfer to the oven and cook, uncovered, for 2–2½ hours, or until the sauce is thick and jammy and the chicken is falling off the bone. Remove the lemon rind before serving.

Fregola salad with herbs

Perfect for a summer barbecue. The more herbs the better, and not just because of the amazing taste: herbs and spices are the richest sources of polyphenols so your gut microbes will thank you.

Prep time: 10 minutes
Cook time: 10 minutes
Serves 2

150g fregola
60g mix of soft herbs (any combination of parsley, mint, chives, tarragon, coriander, basil)
juice of 1 lemon
1 tbsp Dijon mustard
2 tbsp olive oil
salt and pepper

1. Bring a medium saucepan of salted water to the boil and cook the fregola for 10–12 minutes, or until al dente. Drain, rinse under cold water to cool and set aside in a sieve to allow any excess water to drip off while you prepare the herbs.
2. Trim any tough stalks from your herbs and, if using mint, pick the leaves from the stalks. Bunch the herbs together and finely chop.
3. Transfer to a bowl along with the fregola, lemon juice, Dijon mustard, olive oil and a generous pinch of salt and pepper. Mix well to combine and serve.

Fresh tomato spaghetti

Bright, vibrant, silky spaghetti that screams summer.

Prep time: 5 minutes
Cook time: 50 minutes
Serves 2

70ml olive oil
3 garlic cloves, peeled and halved
600g cherry tomatoes
½ tsp sugar (optional)
1 tsp sea salt
1 tsp black pepper
250g spaghetti pasta
Parmesan or pecorino, for serving

1. Pour the olive oil into a medium saucepan, add the garlic, and sauté for 1 minute.
2. Carefully add the tomatoes, sugar, salt and pepper. Place a lid on top and give the pan a vigorous shake to coat the tomatoes in the oil. Simmer on a low heat for 40 minutes, or until the tomatoes have softened and broken down, stirring halfway through.
3. When ready, allow the sauce to cool a little and blitz with a stick blender until smooth. Check for seasoning once more and add salt as needed.
4. Bring a large pot of water to the boil. Add an overly generous pinch of salt and cook the pasta for 10–12 minutes or until al dente. Drain, reserving 2–3 tablespoons of the pasta water.
6. Pour the sauce over the pasta and toss to coat. Add a splash of pasta water, if needed, to loosen. Adorn with plenty of finely grated Parmesan or pecorino cheese and

a drizzle of extra virgin olive oil, and serve with a crisp green salad and bread for mopping.

Fried courgette with white wine vinegar and mint

I love, love, love this recipe. Sweet, fresh and a little sour, it's perfect served with some good bread or with pasta or fish.

Prep time: 8–10 minutes, plus 10 minutes for marinating
Cook time: 25 minutes
Serves 2

4 tbsp olive oil
3 courgettes, sliced into ½cm rounds
1 garlic clove, peeled and finely chopped
3 tbsp white wine vinegar
3 sprigs of mint, leaves picked and finely chopped
salt

1. Place 2 tablespoons of the olive oil in a large frying pan over a medium heat. Add the courgettes with a pinch of salt and sauté for 20–25 minutes, or until they have softened and started to caramelise. Stir in the garlic a few minutes before the end of cooking.
2. Mix the vinegar with the rest of the olive oil to make a dressing.
3. Transfer the courgettes into a small deep dish, and cover with the dressing. Stir in the mint leaves, season and cover with some foil. Allow to marinate for 10 minutes and serve.

Strawberries with honeyed nuts, thyme and lemon

Toasted, sweet nuts, macerated strawberries, thick Greek yoghurt... what more could you want? Remember to buy full-fat yoghurt that contains live bacteria – a probiotic that is great for your gut health.

Prep time: 10 minutes
Cook time: 8 minutes
Serves 2

350g strawberries, quartered
1 tbsp caster sugar
zest of 1 lemon and juice of half
160g mix of pecan and walnuts
3 tbsp honey
2 sprigs of thyme, leaves picked (plus extra to garnish)
200g Greek yoghurt

1. Toss the strawberries with the caster sugar and lemon juice. Set aside to macerate.
2. Preheat the oven to 190°C/170°C fan/gas mark 5. Toss the nuts with the honey, lemon zest and thyme leaves and lay out on a baking tray lined with baking parchment.
3. Roast in the oven for 8 minutes, stirring halfway through, until golden. When ready, remove from the tray immediately (otherwise they will stick) and transfer to a chopping board. When cool, roughly chop.
4. Divide the yoghurt between two bowls, top with strawberries, their juice and the nuts. Garnish with some extra leaves of thyme.

AUTUMN

Mackerel with pickled beetroot

The fatty saltiness of the mackerel and the sour-sweet tang of the pickled beetroot make an ideal combination. Serve with fresh sourdough and a baby leaf salad.

Prep time: 25 minutes
Serves 2

½ tbsp sugar
½ tbsp salt
6 tbsp red wine vinegar
1 medium beetroot, peeled, cut in half and thinly sliced
2 cooked smoked mackerel fillets, skin removed
2 sprigs of dill, finely chopped (optional)
extra-virgin olive oil, to serve
salt and pepper

1. Stir together the sugar and salt in a bowl with 2 tablespoons of boiling-hot water. Once they have dissolved, add the red wine vinegar. Put the sliced beetroot in the bowl, making sure it is fully submerged in the pickling liquid. Set aside for a minimum of 20 minutes.
2. Drain the beetroot and divide it between two plates. Lay the mackerel alongside, top with the dill (if using) and a drizzle of extra-virgin olive oil. Serve with fresh sourdough and a baby leaf salad.

Chilli and garlic greens and beans

This simple dish is packed with flavour and goodness – a perfect emblem of blue-zone cooking.

Prep time: 5 minutes
Cook time: 25 minutes
Serves 2

200g cavolo nero, sliced
100g seasonal greens, sliced (you can use any greens that are in season: spring greens, spinach, mustard greens or a mixture)
4 tbsp olive oil
5 garlic cloves, peeled and finely sliced
½ tsp chilli flakes (or more if you like it spicy)
1 tin cannellini beans, drained and rinsed
100ml chicken or vegetable stock
20g Parmesan, finely grated
juice of ½ lemon
good quality sea salt

1. Remove any tough stalks from the greens and cavolo nero and boil in a large pan of salted water until fully tender – about 15 minutes. Drain and set aside.
2. Sauté the garlic in a large frying pan with 3 tablespoons of the olive oil and after a couple of minutes add the chilli and the drained beans and cook for 3 more minutes.
3. Add in the cooked greens, a splash of water, salt and mix. Cook for a couple of minutes.
4. Stir in the Parmesan and lemon juice and serve with a generous drizzle of extra virgin olive oil and some crunchy sea salt. If you like things spicy, try chilli oil.

Peperonata

Peppers, when slow-fried with tomatoes in a pan, go from bland and boring to deep, sweet umami. I like them with a crispy fried egg on top for breakfast, but you can eat them with pretty much anything.

Prep time: 5 minutes
Cook time: 50 minutes
Serves 2

4 tbsp olive oil
4 large peppers (ideally a mix of red, green and yellow), deseeded and cut into strips
1 onion, peeled and cut into thin strips
5 garlic cloves, peeled and halved
4 medium tomatoes, roughly chopped
splash of red wine vinegar
handful of parsley, chopped
salt

1. Heat the oil in a large saucepan, add the peppers and a pinch of salt, and cook for 5 minutes before adding the onion and garlic. Sauté over a medium heat for 20–30 minutes, or until the veg is beginning to caramelise.
2. Stir in the tomatoes, and season with a pinch of salt. Reduce the heat slightly, cover with a lid and cook slowly for 20 minutes. Add a splash of red wine vinegar at the end and serve with fresh parsley on top.

Chickpea, feta and dill filo pie

I'm obsessed with filo pies and this one is exemplary. I love the contrast of soft bits and crunchy bits. Chickpeas are a great source of fibre, feta is a probiotic (which means it contains microbes that help your gut health), dill is packed with polyphenols and extra virgin olive oil has countless health benefits, including being a powerful anti-inflammatory. All of that in a flakey pie? Heavenly.

Prep time: 20 minutes
Cook time: 1hour
Serves 6–8

2 x 400g tins chickpeas, drained and rinsed
100g dill, finely chopped
25g parsley, chopped
200g feta, crumbled
zest of 3 lemons and juice of 1
3 tsp sea salt
1 tsp freshly ground black pepper
3 tsp tahini
2 cloves garlic, finely chopped
150ml olive oil
9 sheets of filo pastry, kept under a damp tea towel until needed

1. Preheat the oven to 200°C/180°C fan/gas mark 6 and line a 30 x 20cm baking tin with baking parchment.
2. Put the chickpeas in the bowl of a food processor and blitz for a few seconds only – they should appear roughly chopped, not puréed. It is fine for some to be left whole.

Transfer to a large bowl and add the dill, parsley, feta, lemon zest and juice, salt, pepper, tahini, garlic and half the olive oil. Mix well and set aside.

3. Place a sheet of filo in the baking tin – it should be big enough to line the sides as well as the base. Brush all over with olive oil. Repeat with three more sheets of filo, brushing each with olive oil.

4. Spoon one third of the chickpea mixture into the pie base and spread out in an even layer. Brush another sheet of filo with olive oil and this time, fold it in half. Lay it on top of the chickpeas. It should be just the right size to fully cover them. Spoon another layer of chickpeas on top, followed by another sheet of filo.

5. Add the remaining chickpeas into the tin. You should have 3 sheets of filo left. Brush each one with olive oil, fold them in half and lay them on top of the pie.

6. Fold any excess pieces of pastry from the base layers over the top to encase everything. Press down firmly to make sure the pie holds together tightly. Brush the surface with the remaining olive oil and season with some freshly ground black pepper.

7. Bake in the oven for 20 minutes, then reduce the heat to 180°C/160°C fan/gas mark 4 and bake for a further 30–40 minutes, or until the pie is crisp and golden. To check if the underneath is cooked, carefully lift up one side of the pie using a utensil. Once done, remove from the oven, splash a few drops of water on the top of the pie and cover with a clean tea towel. Allow to cool in the tin for at least 30 minutes before slicing.

Caraway and chilli braised baby gem

Cooked lettuce is such an underrated thing. It becomes sweet and comforting and here with caraway seeds and chilli is truly special.

Prep time: 5 minutes
Cook time: 15–20 minutes
Serves 4 as a side

5 tbsp olive oil
4 baby gem lettuce, halved
1 shallot, peeled and finely sliced
1 garlic clove, peeled and finely sliced
½ tsp caraway seeds
½ tsp chilli flakes
150ml white wine
150ml vegetable or chicken stock

1. Place the largest frying pan you have on a high heat with a few tablespoons of olive oil. When the pan is hot, add the lettuce and cook until slightly browned on all sides. It only takes a few minutes and you may need to do it in batches. Add more olive oil as needed. When ready, set aside.
2. Reduce the heat, add some more olive oil so that the pan is coated and stir in the shallot and a pinch of salt. Sauté for 7–8 minutes, then add the garlic and cook for 1 minute longer.
3. Stir in the caraway seeds and chilli flakes, return the lettuce to the pan and pour in the wine. Increase the heat to medium so that the wine is bubbling and cook for about 2 minutes, until it has reduced slightly.

4. Add the stock and cook for 6–8 minutes longer, turning the baby gem over from time to time. The braising liquid will reduce and thicken and become silky with the olive oil. Add the lemon juice and some black pepper if needed. When ready, serve covered with the reduced braising stock.

Mushroomy bolognese

This is my go-to bolognese recipe, one that my family has been making for years. I used to make it with 500g of meat but now I swap half of that for delicious mushrooms and it tastes just as good.

Prep time: 15 minutes
Cook time: 4 hrs 45 minutes
Serves 4–5

5–6 tbsp olive oil
1 onion, peeled and finely diced
2 celery sticks, finely diced
1 large carrot, peeled and finely diced
100g pancetta, diced
500g chestnut mushrooms (or any kind), sliced
250g mix of beef and pork mince
2 tbsp tomato purée
3 garlic cloves, peeled and finely chopped
250ml red wine
400g tin chopped tomatoes
500g pasta
salt and pepper

1. Pour 2 tablespoons of olive oil into a heavy-bottomed casserole dish and sauté the onion for 3–4 minutes. Stir in the carrot and celery, season with a little salt and pepper and sweat the vegetable mix for 8–10 minutes.
2. While this is cooking, place a pan on a medium heat and fry the pancetta in a drizzle of olive oil for about 5 minutes, or until golden brown. Remove with a slotted spoon and set aside. Add the mushrooms to the hot fat

and fry in two batches with a pinch of salt and pepper (adding a little more olive oil if needed) until they have softened and taken on some colour – roughly 5–7 minutes per batch. Remove from the pan and set aside with the pancetta.

3. Add the beef and pork to the pan and cook for 4–5 minutes until browned, then remove from the heat. Set aside the meat with the mushrooms and pancetta. You won't need the frying pan again.

4. In the casserole dish, make a space in the centre of the cooked vegetable mixture, and add the tomato purée. Let that sizzle a little before stirring it through the veg. Add the garlic and cook for 1–2 minutes.

5. Tip the pancetta, mushrooms and meat into the casserole dish and give everything a good stir. Turn the heat up, pour in the wine and simmer vigorously for a few minutes to burn off the alcohol.

6. Add the tomatoes, fill the empty tin with water and pour that in, along with a generous pinch of salt and pepper, and mix well. Turn down the heat, put the lid on and cook for a minimum of 4 hours.

7. Serve with pasta (penne, rigatoni or something similar).

Tip
This bolognese tastes even better if you leave it overnight and reheat it the next day.

Pasta e fagioli

Sticky, slightly spicy and ultra-comforting, this is somewhere between a pasta dish and a soup, and is so much more than the sum of its parts. The ultimate peasant food and very nutritious.

Prep time: 10 minutes
Cook time: 40 minutes
Serves 2

3 tbsp olive oil
1 red onion, peeled and finely chopped
1 carrot, finely diced
1 celery stick, peeled and finely diced
½ tsp chilli flakes
2 cloves garlic, finely chopped
400g tin butter beans, drained and rinsed
200ml passata
handful of fresh parsley
Parmesan rind
400ml water
100g linguini, snapped in half
Parmesan, for serving

1. Heat the olive oil in a casserole dish and gently fry the onion, carrot, celery and a pinch of salt for 15 minutes, stirring often till cooked all the way through. Add a little more oil if necessary.
2. Stir in the chilli flakes, garlic and butter beans and cook for 5 minutes, before adding the passata, parsley and Parmesan rind.
3. Turn up the heat. and stir in 200ml of water from a

boiled kettle and a bit more salt. Add the pasta and stir continuously to release the starch, which will make the sauce thick and creamy.

4. As the pasta absorbs water, top up with the remaining 200ml from the kettle bit by bit, as you could with a risotto. When it is cooked – about 20 minutes – turn off the heat.

5. Serve in shallow bowls with a drizzle of olive oil and a generous helping of Parmesan.

Ricotta with figs, nuts and honey

This is something my nonna and her sisters would be given to eat as a sweet treat when young. Ripe figs are unbeatable. If you can buy locally produced honey, even better.

Prep time: 10 minutes
Serves 2

25g pistachios, roughly chopped
25g blanched hazelnuts, roughly chopped
160g ricotta
2 medium ripe figs, sliced
3 tbsp honey

1. Dry roast the nuts in a small frying pan for a few minutes, and set aside.
2. Beat the ricotta until smooth and divide between two bowls. Top with the figs, nuts and a drizzle of honey.

Orzo with squash and kale

A really scrummy autumnal dish that will have whoever you're feeding asking for seconds. The roast squash will keep for three days in the fridge so you can use what remains in another recipe (see the pumpkin fritters on page 214).

Prep time: 10 minutes
Cook time: 1 hr 15 minutes
Serves 4

½ butternut squash, seeds scooped out
3 tbsp olive oil
1 shallot, peeled and finely chopped
2 garlic cloves, peeled and finely chopped
3 sprigs of rosemary, leaves picked and finely chopped
250g orzo
100ml white wine
750ml chicken or vegetable stock
100g kale, finely sliced
50g Parmesan, grated
salt and pepper

1. Preheat the oven to 200°C/180°C fan/gas mark 6. Put the butternut squash on a large sheet of foil, drizzle with 1 tablespoon of olive oil and a generous pinch of salt and pepper. Wrap the foil around the squash and roast in the oven for 45–50 minutes, or until it is soft when pierced with a knife.
2. Heat 2 tablespoons of olive oil in a medium frying pan and sauté the shallot with a pinch of salt for 5–7 minutes. Add the garlic and rosemary and cook for 1 minute more.

3. Pour in the orzo, increase the heat slightly and toast for 2–3 minutes until it is starting to turn golden.
4. Add the wine and let it bubble vigorously on the high heat for a minute, stirring. Pour in the stock, bring to the boil and then reduce the heat to a simmer. Cover with a lid and cook for 10 minutes.
5. Scoop the squash from its skin and mash until smooth. Add this to the orzo, along with the kale and Parmesan. Mix everything together and cook for 1–2 minutes, then remove from the heat. Place the lid back on top and allow the orzo to rest for 2–3 minutes and the kale to further soften. Serve with an extra drizzle of olive oil.

Butterbean and mushroom stew with chestnuts and thyme

Fantastically tasty and packed with goodness. My top tip is to seek out the best beans you can – I find that the ones in jars tend to be of higher quality than ones in cans. My favourite is by Bold Bean Co. If you're using these don't wash away the bean stock – it provides vital flavour so add it all into your stew.

Prep time: 15 minutes
Cook time: 50 minutes
Serves 4

40g dried porcini mushrooms
450g chestnut mushrooms, finely sliced
5 tbsp olive oil
1 leek, finely sliced
½ onion, peeled and finely chopped
2 garlic cloves, peeled and finely chopped
5 sprigs thyme, leaves picked
1½ tbsp flour
400ml chicken or vegetable stock
400g tin butter beans, drained and rinsed
180g cooked chestnuts, roughly chopped
20g parsley, roughly chopped
juice of ½ lemon

1. Put the dried mushrooms in a bowl or jug and cover with 200ml of boiling hot water.
2. Place a wide casserole dish on a high heat with 2 tablespoons of olive oil and fry the chestnut mushrooms for 6–8 minutes, until softened and golden. Transfer to a bowl.

3. Add the remaining oil to the pan, reduce the heat and fry the onion and leek with a pinch of salt for 10–12 minutes, stirring occasionally. Add the garlic and thyme and cook for 1 minute more.

4. Stir in the flour and cook for a few seconds. Drain the dried mushrooms and finely chop, then add these to the pan, along with the mushroom stock, chicken stock, butter beans, chestnuts and the fried chestnut mushrooms. Simmer for 30 minutes.

5. Remove from the heat, stir in the parsley and lemon juice and serve.

White wine braised fennel

Simple and stunning. Serve this sweet, aniseed veggie alongside roast chicken, pork or fish or eat with some lovely fresh bread and cheese.

Prep time: 5 minutes
Cook time: 45 minutes
Serves 2

2 tbsp olive oil
3 fennel bulbs, trimmed and sliced in 6 lengthways
2 garlic cloves, peeled and cut in half
½ lemon, sliced in half
50ml white wine
salt and pepper

1. Heat the olive oil in a large casserole dish (one with a tight-fitting lid). Add the fennel and cook on a medium heat for 5–7 minutes or until starting to take on some colour.
2. Reduce the heat to low and add the garlic, lemon, white wine and a generous pinch of salt and pepper to the pan. Mix together, cover with a sheet of baking parchment, followed by the lid, and cook on a low heat for 40 minutes.

Blackberry and orange olive oil pudding

This delicious pudding is so simple to make. And the olive oil is a winner – trust me.

Prep time: 10 minutes
Cook time: 50 minutes
Serves 4–6

70ml olive oil
225 ml whole milk
150g spelt or plain flour
185g plus 1 tbsp caster sugar
1 tsp baking powder
zest of 1 orange
180g frozen blackberries

1. Preheat the oven to 180°C/160°C fan/gas mark 4 and line a round baking tin with baking parchment.
2. Put the olive oil, milk, flour, sugar, baking powder and orange zest in a bowl and mix until smooth. Pour into the prepared tin and scatter the frozen berries all over.
3. Drizzle 1 tablespoon of sugar all over the surface and bake in the oven for 45–50 minutes, or until a skewer inserted comes out clean.

Tip
Using frozen berries is crucial otherwise the cake will be soggy.

WINTER

Root vegetable soup with barley

Barley with its nubbly texture is so good in soups and works perfectly here with the flavour-infused root veg.

Prep time: 15 minutes
Cook time: 45 minutes
Serves 4

3 tbsp olive oil
1 onion, peeled and roughly chopped
3 carrots, peeled and cut into 2cm dice
2 celery sticks, roughly diced
4 sprigs of thyme, leaves picked
1 garlic clove, peeled and roughly chopped
1 small celeriac, peeled and cut into 2cm dice
2 parsnips, peeled and cut into 2cm dice
70g pearl barley
1.5 litres chicken stock

1. Place the olive oil, onion, carrot, celery and thyme in a large saucepan that has a lid. Add a pinch of salt and sweat the vegetables for 10 minutes on a low heat, stirring occasionally. Stir in the garlic and cook for 1 minute more.
2. Add the remaining vegetables, pearl barley and stock. Bring to a simmer and cook with the lid on for 30–40 minutes, until the vegetables and barley are tender. Season to taste and serve.

Slow-cooked leeks with lemon and walnuts

This is so easy to make and the result is sensational. Soft, sweet, lemony leeks with the crumbly crunch of walnuts. Great as a side, or mixed through pasta.

Prep time: 10 minutes
Cook time: 40 minutes
Serves 2 as a main, 4 as a side

2 large leeks (roughly 500g), cut into ½cm slices
zest and juice of 1 lemon
5 sprigs of thyme, leaves picked
3 tbsp olive oil
salt and pepper
7 sprigs of parsley, leaves picked and roughly chopped
60g walnuts, toasted in a dry frying pan

1. Place the leeks, lemon zest and juice, thyme, olive oil and some seasoning in a saucepan with a tight-fitting lid and cook slowly for 35–40 minutes, stirring from time to time.
2. When ready, stir in the parsley and a pinch of salt and serve topped with toasted walnuts.

Pumpkin fritters with salsa verde

Salsa verde is a fantastic way to use up leftover herbs in your fridge. As long as you have a base of parsley, you can use any combination of soft herbs. Try these fritters as a snack, or as part of a main meal, or even for breakfast with an egg.

Prep time: 15 minutes
Cook time: 12–15 minutes
Makes 8 fritters

For the fritters:
½ small butternut squash, coarsely grated
50g Parmesan, coarsely grated
3 sprigs of sage or rosemary, leaves picked and finely chopped
1 egg
1½ tsp baking powder
35g flour
1 tbsp olive oil

For the salsa verde:
½ garlic clove, peeled
20g parsley, roughly chopped
20g mix of mint, basil, dill, chives and/or tarragon
zest and juice of ½ lemon
3 tbsp olive oil
½ tbsp red wine vinegar
½ tbsp Dijon mustard
½ tbsp capers
2 cornichons (or a few extra capers)

1. First make the salsa verde. Place all the ingredients in a food processor and pulse until the herbs are roughly chopped. Season with salt and pepper and set aside.

2. Put all of the ingredients for the fritters (except the olive oil) into a bowl and mix until combined. Season with a pinch of salt and pepper. With damp hands, shape the mixture into 8 fritters. You can make this recipe up to this point and refrigerate until needed.

3. Place a large frying pan on a medium heat with the olive oil. When hot, fry the fritters for 3–4 minutes on each side, until golden and crisp. Turn the heat down slightly if necessary. You may need to cook the fritters in two batches.

4. When ready, serve with the salsa verde. A simple green salad alongside is lovely too.

Bitter leaf salad with burrata, pears and walnuts

The most delicious combination. If you can't find burrata then mozzarella works well too.

Prep time: 10 minutes
Serves 2

50g walnuts
1 pear
juice of ½ lemon
100g mix of bitter leaves, such as radicchio/frisée/chicory
1 ball of burrata
3 tbsp olive oil
1½ tbsp balsamic vinegar

1. Toast the walnuts in a dry frying pan for 2–3 minutes until golden and fragrant. Transfer to a chopping board and when cool, roughly chop.
2. Thinly slice the pear and dress with lemon juice to stop it from going brown.
3. Divide the leaves between two bowls, drizzle the olive oil all over and season. Place the pear and chopped walnuts on top. Tear the burrata into pieces and lay on top of the salad. Finish with the balsamic, season once more and serve.

Onion and herb frittata

The trick here is to cook the onions gently and slowly until they're sweet and very soft. A great portable lunch.

Prep time: 10 minutes
Cook time: 30 minutes
Serves 2

2 medium onions, peeled and finely sliced
2 tbsp olive oil
30g parsley, finely chopped
5 medium free-range eggs
salt and pepper

1. Place the onions, olive oil and a pinch of salt in a medium non-stick frying pan (approx. 22cm diameter) and sauté on a low heat, stirring occasionally, for 25–30 minutes, or until golden brown and beginning to caramlise. Allow to cool slightly.
2. In a bowl or jug, whisk the eggs with the parsley and a generous pinch of salt and pepper. Stir in the cooled onions. Turn your grill to high.
3. Return the pan to a low heat (no need to wash it) and pour in the egg mixture. Cook for 4–5 minutes, or until it is golden brown underneath and the edges are starting to become crispy.
4. Place the pan under the hot grill for 1 minute, by which time the frittata should have set. Tip it out onto a serving plate and serve on its own or with a green salad.

Tip
If you are using a smaller frying pan, the frittata will be thicker so leave it under the grill for a few minutes more.

Caramelised cauliflower, onion and garlic dip

Move over hummus, there's a new dip in town. This is phenomenal on toasted bread, alongside salad or as a condiment for chicken. To be honest, it's good enough to eat on its own.

Prep time: 10 minutes
Cook time: 50 minutes
Makes 360g

½ medium cauliflower (roughly 350g), stalks included, roughly chopped
1 medium onion, peeled and roughly chopped
4 garlic cloves, peeled
5 sprigs of thyme, leaves picked
4 tbsp olive oil
salt and pepper

1. Preheat the oven to 180°C/160°C fan/gas mark 4. Place the cauliflower, onion, garlic and thyme in a small roasting tin, toss with the olive oil and season with salt and pepper.
2. Roast in the oven for 40–50 minutes or until browned and slightly caramelised.
3. Allow to cool a little, then transfer to a food processor and blend until smooth. Refrigerate until needed.

New Year's Day lentil soup

Full of protein, fibre and nutrients and very affordable, lentils are a great addition to your diet. This soup shows you how delicious they can be too.

Prep time: 15 minutes
Cook time: 50 minutes
Serves 4

3 tbsp olive oil
1 onion, peeled and finely chopped
2 medium carrots, peeled and finely chopped
2 celery sticks, finely chopped
2 garlic cloves, peeled and roughly chopped
200g puy lentils
400g tin chopped tomatoes
1.4 litres stock (meat, chicken or vegetable)
2 sprigs of thyme
2 sprigs of rosemary
250g cavolo nero, tough stems removed and roughly chopped
salt and pepper
Parmesan, lemon juice and best-quality olive oil, to finish

1. Pour the olive oil into a large saucepan (one with a lid) over a medium heat and sauté the onion, carrots and celery with a pinch of salt for 10 minutes or until softened. Add the garlic and cook for 1 minute more.
2. Stir the lentils into the mixture, along with the chopped tomatoes and another pinch of salt. Add the stock, stir in the herbs and bring to the boil.

3. Reduce to a gentle simmer, cover with a lid and cook for 30 minutes.
4. Stir the cavolo nero into the soup and cook for another 10 minutes. Season to taste. Ladle into bowls and finish with grated Parmesan, a squeeze of lemon and a drizzle of olive oil.

Tip
This soup will keep for 4–5 days in the fridge and actually tastes better with every passing day. It also freezes well.

Chicory with herbs, chilli and lemon

Charring the chicory is key here for maximum flavour and I just adore the golden breadcrumbs on the top.

Prep time: 10 minutes
Cook time: 30 minutes
Serves 2

4 heads of chicory, sliced in 4 lengthways
5 sprigs of dill, finely chopped
zest and juice of 1 lemon
½ tsp chilli flakes
pinch of sugar
50ml olive oil, plus 1 tbsp extra
salt and pepper
50g breadcrumbs (from good-quality bread such as sourdough)

1. Preheat the oven to 180°C/160°C fan/gas mark 4. Lay the chicory in a single layer on a baking tray.
2. In a small bowl, mix together the dill, lemon zest and juice, chilli flakes, sugar, salt and pepper, along with 50ml olive oil. Spoon over the chicory, making sure it is all evenly coated.
3. Bake in the oven for 30 minutes, or until the chicory has softened and the edges are slightly charred (it should still have a little bit of bite).
4. Meanwhile, pour the remaining tablespoon of olive oil into a medium frying pan and fry the breadcrumbs over a medium heat for 2–3 minutes, or until golden and crisp. Season with a pinch of salt and pepper.
5. When the chicory is ready, scatter over the breadcrumbs and serve.

Mushroom broth with chicken and garlic

The star of the show in this recipe are the mushrooms, with the chicken just enhancing the flavour. A deep, nourishing and unique dish with the addition of wonderful juniper berries.

Prep time: 10 minutes
Cook time: 1 hr 20 minutes
Serves 2

1 chicken thigh or leg, skin on and bone in
2 tbsp olive oil
2 shallots, peeled and finely sliced
4 sprigs of thyme, leaves picked
3 sprigs of rosemary, leaves picked and finely chopped
3 garlic cloves, peeled and roughly chopped
500g portobello mushrooms, sliced
750ml vegetable or chicken stock
5 juniper berries
juice of ½ lemon
salt and pepper

1. Heat the olive oil in a medium saucepan. Salt the chicken, add to the pan and brown on all sides until the skin is golden and some of the fat has been rendered off. Remove and set aside.
2. Reduce the heat and add the shallots, thyme and rosemary with a pinch of salt. Sauté for 7–8 minutes, until softened. Add the garlic and cook for 1 minute more.
3. Put the mushrooms into the saucepan and stir to coat with the oil. Place a tight fitting lid on top and cook for about 7 minutes, stirring occasionally. The mushrooms will reduce in size and give up their delicious juices.

4. Add the browned chicken to the saucepan along with the chicken stock and juniper berries. Bring to the boil and then reduce the heat so that it is very gently simmering. Cover with a lid and cook for 1 hour.

5. When ready, remove the juniper berries if you can find them! They usually float on the surface. Shred the meat from the chicken (discard the skin and bone) and return to the broth. Add the lemon juice and season to taste with salt and pepper.

Borlotti bean, squash and chard stew

A hearty winter stew given richness and depth by the addition of red wine. The sweet squash and slightly bitter chard are the best companions.

Prep time: 15 minutes
Cook time: 2hrs 15 minutes
Serves 6

7 tbsp olive oil
1 onion, peeled and finely chopped
2 carrots, peeled and finely diced
2 celery sticks, finely diced
4 garlic cloves, peeled and finely chopped
4 sprigs of thyme, leaves picked
3 sprigs of rosemary, leaves picked and finely chopped
2 tbsp tomato purée
2 tbsp flour
300ml red wine
400g tin chopped tomatoes
800ml chicken or vegetable stock
2 400g tins borlotti beans, drained and rinsed
1 butternut squash, halved, seeds scooped out and each half cut into 6
200g chard, finely shredded

1. Preheat the oven to 150°C/130°C fan/ gas mark 2. Heat 5 tablespoons of olive oil in a large casserole dish and add the onion, carrots, celery and a generous pinch of salt. Stir and place a lid on top and sweat the soffritto mix for 10 minutes on a low heat. Add the herbs and garlic and cook for 2 minutes more.

2. Make a well in the centre and cook the tomato purée for 1 minute or so. Stir in the flour until it is coating the vegetables and cook for 1 minute more.

3. Increase the heat and add the wine. Simmer to cook off some of the alcohol and until the flour has thickened the sauce – 2 minutes or so. Pour in the chopped tomatoes, stock and borlotti beans. Season again with salt and pepper, mix to combine and bring to the boil. Place the lid on top and transfer to the oven for 1 hour 50 minutes.

4. Lay the butternut squash in a roasting dish and drizzle the remaining olive oil all over. Season with salt and pepper, and place in the oven for the same amount of time as the casserole.

5. Remove both dishes from the oven. Carefully remove the lid of the casserole dish and stir in the chard. Submerge the squash into the stew also, place the lid on top and return to the oven for 10 minutes. Check for seasoning, adding a touch more salt or pepper if needed and serve.

Thyme and lemon poached pears

These poached pears are aromatic, fragrant and sweet. My advice is to make them the night before you plan to serve them and allow them to infuse as the poaching liquid cools.

Prep time: 10 minutes
Cook time: 40–50 minutes
Serves 4

2 unwaxed lemons
150ml honey
150g golden caster sugar
10g bunch of thyme
10 peppercorns
crème fraîche and wedge of lemon, to serve

1. Peel the rind from both lemons and place in a large saucepan. Add the juice of one lemon and slice the other into ½cm slices, removing the pips. Put these in the pan also.
2. Add the honey, caster sugar, thyme and peppercorns and cover with 800ml water.
3. Slowly bring to the boil, stirring to dissolve the sugar. Reduce the heat to low so that the syrup is gently simmering.
4. Add the pears and place a piece of parchment on top. Poach for 30-40 minutes – they should be tender when pierced with a knife. Underripe pears may take longer.
5. When ready, remove from the stock with a slotted spoon and serve with a dollop of crème fraîche, some of the poaching syrup and a squeeze of lemon juice.

Tip
When you have served the pears, strain the poaching liquid and reduce by half until it is thick and syrupy. Store in the fridge for 2–3 weeks and spoon over yoghurt or ice cream, or use as a cordial to make a delicious drink.

Best chicken stock

Having a good stock ready for use in the fridge is key to blue-zone cooking. This recipe gives you the cornerstones of a great one, so much better than any stock you can buy.

Prep time: 10 minutes
Cook time: 2½ hours
Makes 1½–2 litres

1kg chicken wings
2 tbsp olive oil
1 onion, peeled and studded with 4 cloves
1 leek, cut into chunks
3 carrots, cut into chunks
3 celery sticks, cut into chunks
4 garlic cloves
handful of thyme and/or rosemary
1 bay leaf
1 tomato, quartered
rind of Parmesan, if you have one
salt and pepper

1. In a very large pot, brown off the chicken wings in the olive oil so that their skin is slightly golden.
2. Add the rest of the ingredients and cover with 3 litres of water. Bring to the boil and then reduce the heat so that the stock is gently simmering. Skim off any scum that rises to the surface and continue to do this throughout the cooking time.
3. Cover with a lid and simmer for 2½ hours. Either leave the stock overnight to infuse further before straining, or strain immediately and season to taste.

4. If not being used immediately, the stock will keep for 4–5 days in the fridge or can be frozen. You can also reduce the stock by half for a stronger, more intense flavour – just remember to season the stock *after* you have reduced it!

Slow-cooked beef with thyme, garlic and brown lentils

A phenomenal winter dish, deep and unctuous with slow-cooked meat and earthy lentils. Brilliant with some simply cooked green veg.

Prep time: 15 minutes
Cook time: 2hrs 30 minutes
Serves 4

300g shin of beef (bone in)
1 tbsp white flour
4 tbsp olive oil
1 medium onion, peeled and sliced
2 medium carrots, peeled and cut into 3cm chunks
2 celery sticks, cut into 2cm dice
4 garlic cloves, peeled and sliced
500ml red wine
900ml beef stock
200g brown lentils
8 sprigs of thyme
20g Parmesan, finely grated
1 tsp red wine vinegar
salt and pepper

1. Preheat the oven to 150°C/130°C fan/gas mark 2. Toss the beef in the flour and season with a generous pinch of salt and pepper. Heat 1 tablespoon of the oil in a large casserole dish, brown the shin on both sides and set aside.
2. Add the remaining oil to the pan with the onion, carrots and celery. Sweat with a lid on for 10 minutes, stirring occasionally. Add the garlic and cook for 1 minute more.

3. Pour in the wine and increase the heat slightly. Simmer for a minute or so to burn off some of the alcohol. Return the beef to the pan, add the beef stock, lentils and thyme. Bring to a simmer, cover with a lid and transfer to the oven for 2–2½ hours, or until the beef is meltingly tender and the lentils are soft.

4. When you are ready to serve, remove the thyme sprigs from the stew and shred the beef from the bone. Add the Parmesan, plus a pinch of salt and pepper if needed, and stir in the red wine vinegar to bring all the flavours to life.

Endnotes

1 Our World in Data. (2023) *Life expectancy in males and females, World.* ourworldindata.org

2 World Health Organization. (2019) 'World Health Statistics 2019: Monitoring health for the Sdgs, Sustainable Development Goals'.

3 Herskind, A.M. et al. (1996) 'The heritability of human longevity: A population-based study of 2872 Danish twin pairs born 1870–1900,' *Human Genetics*, 97(3), p. 319

4 Buxton, J. (2021) *National life tables – life expectancy in the UK - Office for National Statistics.* ons.gov.uk

5 Buxton, J. (2021) *National life tables – life expectancy in the UK - Office for National Statistics.* ons.gov.uk

6 Kotifani, A. (2024) 'Power 9®,' Blue Zones. bluezones.com/2016/11/power-9/.

7 Fadnes, L.T. et al. (2022) 'Estimating impact of food choices on life expectancy: A modeling study,' *PLOS Medicine*, 19(2), p. e1003889. doi.org/10.1371/journal.pmed.1003889

8 Afshin, A. et al. (2019) 'Health effects of dietary risks in 195 countries, 1990–2017: A systematic analysis for the Global Burden of Disease Study 2017,' *The Lancet*, 393(10184), pp. 1958–1972. doi.org/10.1016/s0140-6736(19)30041-8

9 Mintel. (2021) *Sales of oat milk overtake almond.* mintel.com/press-centre

10 La Berge, A.F. (2007) 'How the deology of low fat conquered America,' *Journal of the History of Medicine and Allied Sciences*, 63(2), pp. 139–177. doi.org/10.1093/jhmas/jrn001

11 Hubert, H.B. et al. (1983) 'Obesity as an independent risk factor for cardiovascular disease: A 26-year follow-up of participants in the Framingham Heart Study', *Circulation*, 67(5), pp. 968–977. doi.org/10.1161/01.cir.67.5.968

12 Tobias, D.K. et al. (2015) 'Effect of low-fat diet interventions versus other diet interventions on long-term weight change in adults: a systematic review and meta-analysis,' *The Lancet Diabetes & Endocrinology*, 3(12), pp. 968–979. doi.org/10.1016/s2213-8587(15)00367-8.

13 Tremblay, A., Doyon, C.Y. and Sánchez, M. (2015) 'Impact of yogurt on appetite control, energy balance, and body composition,' *Nutrition Reviews*, 73(suppl 1), pp. 23–27. doi.org/10.1093/nutrit/nuv015

14 Martínez-González, M.Á., Ros, E. and Estruch, R. (2018) 'Primary prevention of cardiovascular disease with a Mediterranean diet supplemented with extra-virgin olive oil or nuts,' *The New England Journal of Medicine*, 378(25), p. e34. doi.org/10.1056/nejmoa1800389

15 British Heart Foundation. (2021) *Fats explained*. bhf.org.uk

16 Scott, E. (2023) *Mortality rates among men and women: impact of austerity*. lordslibrary.parliament.uk

17 Eurostat. (2019) *Overweight and obesity - BMI statistics*. ec.europa.eu

18 NHS England. (2022) *Health Survey for England, 2021: Data tables - NHS Digital*. digital.nhs.uk/data-and-information

19 The Food Foundation. (2022) *The Broken Plate 2022*. foodfoundation.org.uk

20 Frontier Economics. (2023) *Updated estimates of the cost of obesity and overweightness*. frontier-economics.com

21 Rauber, F. et al. (2019) 'Ultra-processed foods and excessive free sugar intake in the UK: A nationally representative cross-sectional study,' *BMJ Open*, 9(10), p. e027546. doi.org/10.1136/bmjopen-2018-027546

22 Parnham, J.C. et al. (2022) 'The ultra-processed food content of school meals and packed lunches in the UK, 2008–17: A pooled cross-sectional study,' *The Lancet*, 400, p. S12. doi.org/10.1016/s0140-6736(22)02222-x

23 Monteiro, C.A. et al. (2019) 'Ultra-processed foods: what they are and how to identify them,' *Public Health Nutrition*, 22(5), pp. 936–941. doi.org/10.1017/s1368980018003762.

24 Elizabeth, L. et al. (2020) 'Ultra-processed foods and health outcomes: A narrative review,' *Nutrients*, 12(7), p. 1955. doi.org/10.3390/nu12071955

25 The Food Foundation. (2023) *The Broken Plate 2023*. foodfoundation.org.uk

26 NCD Risk Factor Collaboration. *Evolution of height over time*. https://ncdrisc.org/height-mean-map.htm

27 Pes, G.M. et al. (2014) 'Male longevity in Sardinia, a review of historical sources supporting a causal link with dietary factors,' *European Journal of Clinical Nutrition*, 69(4), pp. 411–418. doi.org/10.1038/ejcn.2014.230

28 Buettner, D. (2015) *The blue zones solution: Eating and living like the world's healthiest people*. National Geographic Books.

29 Nieddu, A. et al. (2020) 'Dietary habits, anthropometric features and daily performance in two independent long-lived populations from Nicoya peninsula

(Costa Rica) and Ogliastra (Sardinia),' *Nutrients*, 12(6), p. 1621. doi.org/10.3390/nu12061621

30 Wang, C. et al. (2022) 'Sardinian dietary analysis for longevity: a review of the literature,' *Journal of Ethnic Foods*, 9(1). doi.org/10.1186/s42779-022-00152-5

31 Gillam, S. (2019) 'Do you Bant? The original low-carbohydrate, high-fat (LCHF) diet,' *Royal College of Surgeons*, 13 May. rcseng.ac.uk/library-and-publications/library/blog/do-you-bant/

32 Wanders, A.J. et al. (2011) 'Effects of dietary fibre on subjective appetite, energy intake and body weight: a systematic review of randomized controlled trials,' *Obesity Reviews*, 12(9), pp. 724–739. doi.org/10.1111/j.1467-789x.2011.00895.x

33 Clark, M.J. and Slavin, J.L. (2013) 'The Effect of fiber on satiety and food intake: a systematic review,' *Journal of the American College of Nutrition*, 32(3), pp. 200–211. doi.org/10.1080/07315724.2013.791194.

34 Behall, K.M., Scholfield, D.J. and Hallfrisch, J. (2004) 'Diets containing barley significantly reduce lipids in mildly hypercholesterolemic men and women,' *The American Journal of Clinical Nutrition*, 80(5), pp. 1185–1193. doi.org/10.1093/ajcn/80.5.1185.

35 Ho, H.V.T. et al. (2016) 'A systematic review and meta-analysis of randomized controlled trials of the effect of barley β-glucan on LDL-C, non-HDL-C and apoB for cardiovascular disease risk reductioni-iv,' *European Journal of Clinical Nutrition*, 70(11), pp. 1239–1245. doi.org/10.1038/ejcn.2016.89.

36 Rolim, M.E. et al. (2022) 'Consumption of sourdough bread and changes in the glycemic control and satiety: A systematic review,' *Critical Reviews in Food Science and Nutrition*, pp. 1–16. doi.org/10.1080/10408398.2022.2108756

37 Stamataki, N.S., Yanni, A.E. and Karathanos, V.T. (2017) 'Bread making technology influences postprandial glucose response: a review of the clinical evidence,' *British Journal of Nutrition*, 117(7), pp. 1001–1012. doi.org/10.1017/s0007114517000770

38 Ma, S. et al. (2021) 'Sourdough improves the quality of whole-wheat flour products: Mechanisms and challenges—A review,' *Food Chemistry*, 360, p. 130038. doi.org/10.1016/j.foodchem.2021.130038

39 Willcox, D.C., Scapagnini, G. and Willcox, B.J. (2014) 'Healthy aging diets other than the Mediterranean: A focus on the Okinawan diet,' *Mechanisms of Ageing and Development*, 136–137, pp. 148–162. doi.org/10.1016/j.mad.2014.01.002

40 Willcox B, Willcox D.C. and Suzuki M. (2004) *The Okinawa Diet Plan*. New York: Three Rivers Press.

41 Couteur, D.G.L. et al. (2016) 'New Horizons: dietary protein, ageing and the Okinawan ratio,' *Age and Ageing*, 45(4), pp. 443–447. doi.org/10.1093/ageing/afw069

42 Willcox, B.J., Willcox, D.C. and Suzuki, M. (2017) 'Demographic, phenotypic, and genetic characteristics of centenarians in Okinawa and Japan: Part 1– Centenarians in Okinawa,' *Mechanisms of Ageing and Development*, 165, pp. 75–79. doi.org/10.1016/j.mad.2016.11.001

43 Couteur, D.G.L. et al. (2015) 'The impact of low-protein high-carbohydrate diets on aging and lifespan,' *Cellular and Molecular Life Sciences*, 73(6), pp. 1237–1252. doi.org/10.1007/s00018-015-2120-y

44 Wahl, D. et al. (2018) 'Comparing the effects of low-protein and high-carbohydrate diets and caloric restriction on brain aging in mice,' *Cell Reports*, 25(8), pp. 2234-2243.e6. doi.org/10.1016/j.celrep.2018.10.070

45 Couteur, D.G.L. et al. (2016) 'New Horizons: dietary protein, ageing and the Okinawan ratio,' *Age and Ageing*, 45(4), pp. 443–447. doi.org/10.1093/ageing/afw069

46 Pes, G.M. et al. (2014) 'Male longevity in Sardinia, a review of historical sources supporting a causal link with dietary factors,' *European Journal of Clinical Nutrition*, 69(4), pp. 411–418. doi.org/10.1038/ejcn.2014.230

47 Wang, C. et al. (2022) 'Sardinian dietary analysis for longevity: a review of the literature,' *Journal of Ethnic Foods*, 9(1). doi.org/10.1186/s42779-022-00152-5

48 Nieddu, A. et al. (2020b) 'Dietary habits, anthropometric features and daily performance in two independent long-lived populations from Nicoya peninsula (Costa Rica) and Ogliastra (Sardinia),' *Nutrients*, 12(6), p. 1621. doi.org/10.3390/nu12061621

49 Blue Zones. (2023) *Nicoya, Costa Rica – Blue zones*. bluezones.com/explorations/nicoya-costa-rica/

50 Blue Zones. (2023) *Loma Linda, California – Blue zones* (2022). bluezones.com/explorations/loma-linda-california/

51 Blue Zones. (2023) *Food guidelines*. bluezones.com/recipes/food-guidelines/

52 Siasos, G. et al. (2013) 'Consumption of a boiled Greek type of coffee is associated with improved endothelial function: The Ikaria Study,' *Vascular Medicine*, 18(2), pp. 55–62. doi.org/10.1177/1358863x13480258

53 Hyman, M., MD (2019) *7 Takeaways About Meat from My Book Food: What the Heck Should I Eat?* drhyman.com

54 Farvid, M.S. et al. (2021) 'Consumption of red meat and processed meat and cancer incidence: a systematic review and meta-analysis of prospective studies,' *European Journal of Epidemiology*, 36(9), pp. 937–951. doi.org/10.1007/s10654-021-00741-9

55 Knüppel, A. et al. (2020) 'Meat intake and cancer risk: prospective analyses in UK Biobank,' *International Journal of Epidemiology*, 49(5), pp. 1540–1552. doi.org/10.1093/ije/dyaa142

56 Research Gate. *Mediterranean Diet Adherence Screener.* researchgate.net

57 Bradbury, K.E., Murphy, N. and Key, T.J. (2019) 'Diet and colorectal cancer in UK Biobank: a prospective study,' *International Journal of Epidemiology*, 49(1), pp. 246–258. doi.org/10.1093/ije/dyz064

58 British Nutrition Foundation. (2021) *The science of protein.* nutrition.org.uk.

59 Office for Health Improvement and Disparities (2023) *National Diet and Nutrition Survey.*

60 Mosley, M. (2022) *Dr Michael Mosley: The best way to lose weight? Eat more protein.* sciencefocus.com/the-human-body/dr-michael-mosley-eat-more-protein

61 Raubenheimer, D. and Simpson, S.J. (2023) 'Protein appetite as an integrator in the obesity system: the protein leverage hypothesis,' *Philosophical Transactions of the Royal Society B*, 378(1888). doi.org/10.1098/rstb.2022.0212

62 Seidelmann, S.B. et al. (2018) 'Dietary carbohydrate intake and mortality: a prospective cohort study and meta-analysis,' *The Lancet Public Health*, 3(9), pp. e419–e428. doi.org/10.1016/s2468-2667(18)30135-x

63 Harvard T.H. Chan School of Public Health (2016) *Processed red meat related to higher risk of death, plant protein to lower risk.* hsph.harvard.edu/nutritionsource/2016/08/09/processed-red-meat-higher-risk-of-death-plant-protein-lower-risk/

64 Harvard T. H. Chan School of Public Health (2023). *Protein.* hsph.harvard.edu/nutritionsource/what-should-you-eat/protein/

65 Nieddu, A. et al. (2020) 'Dietary habits, anthropometric features and daily performance in two independent long-lived populations from Nicoya peninsula (Costa Rica) and Ogliastra (Sardinia),' *Nutrients*, 12(6), p. 1621. doi.org/10.3390/nu12061621

66 Zhang, H. et al. (2021) 'Meat consumption and risk of incident dementia: cohort study of 493,888 UK Biobank participants,' *The American Journal of Clinical Nutrition*, 114(1), pp. 175–184. doi.org/10.1093/ajcn/nqab028

67 Provenza, F.D., Kronberg, S.L. and Gregorini, P. (2019) 'Is grassfed meat and

dairy better for human and environmental health?,' *Frontiers in Nutrition*, 6. doi.org/10.3389/fnut.2019.00026

68 Longo, V. (2019) *The longevity diet*. Canada: Penguin Random House.

69 National Geographic. On Beyond 100. nationalgeographic.com

70 Darmadi-Blackberry, I. et al. (2004) 'Legumes: the most important dietary predictor of survival in older people of different ethnicities'. *Asia Pacific Journal of Clinical Nutrition*

71 Chang, W.-S.W. et al. (2011) 'A bean-free diet increases the risk of all-cause mortality among Taiwanese women: the role of the metabolic syndrome,' *Public Health Nutrition*, 15(4), pp. 663–672. doi.org/10.1017/s1368980011002151

72 Kim, S.J. et al. (2016) 'Effects of dietary pulse consumption on body weight: a systematic review and meta-analysis of randomized controlled trials,' The American Journal of Clinical Nutrition, 103(5), pp. 1213–1223. doi.org/10.3945/ajcn.115.124677

73 Kristensen, M.L. et al. (2016) 'Meals based on vegetable protein sources (beans and peas) are more satiating than meals based on animal protein sources (veal and pork) – a randomized cross-over meal test study,' *Food & Nutrition Research*, 60(1), p. 32634. doi.org/10.3402/fnr.v60.32634

74 Papanikolaou, Y. and Fulgoni, V.L. (2008) 'Bean consumption is associated with greater nutrient intake, reduced systolic blood pressure, lower body weight, and a smaller waist circumference in adults: results from the National Health and Nutrition Examination Survey 1999-2002,' *Journal of the American College of Nutrition*, 27(5), pp. 569–576. doi.org/10.1080/07315724.2008.10719740

75 Reister, E.J. and Leidy, H.J. (2020) 'An afternoon hummus snack affects diet quality, appetite, and glycemic control in healthy adults,' *The Journal of Nutrition*, 150(8), pp. 2214–2222. doi.org/10.1093/jn/nxaa139

76 Court, A. (2023) 'Ozempic users report gross side effect: "Join the s--t the bed club," New York Post, 24 May. nypost.com

77 Nilsson, A. et al. (2013) 'Effects of a brown beans evening meal on metabolic risk markers and appetite regulating hormones at a subsequent standardized breakfast: a randomized Cross-Over study,' PLOS ONE, 8(4), p. e59985. doi.org/10.1371/journal.pone.0059985

78 Bielefeld, D., Grafenauer, S. and Rangan, A. (2020) 'The effects of legume consumption on markers of glycaemic control in individuals with and without diabetes mellitus: a systematic literature review of randomised controlled trials,' nutrients, 12(7), p. 2123. doi.org/10.3390/nu12072123

79 Becerra-Tomás, N., Papandreou, C. and Salas-Salvadó, J. (2019) 'Legume consumption and cardiometabolic health,' Advances in Nutrition, 10, pp. S437–S450. doi.org/10.1093/advances/nmz003

80 Messina, V. (2014) 'Nutritional and health benefits of dried beans,' The American Journal of Clinical Nutrition, 100, pp. 437S-442S. doi.org/10.3945/ajcn.113.071472

81 Del Rio, D. et al. (2013) 'Dietary (poly)phenolics in human health: structures, bioavailability, and evidence of protective effects against chronic diseases,' antioxidants & redox signaling, 18(14), pp. 1818–1892. doi.org/10.1089/ars.2012.4581

82 Bao, Y. et al. (2013) 'Association of Nut Consumption with Total and Cause-Specific Mortality,' *The New England Journal of Medicine*, 369(21), pp. 2001–2011. doi.org/10.1056/nejmoa1307352

83 Liu, X., Gausch-Ferré, M., Tobias D. and Li Y. (2021) 'Association of Walnut Consumption with Total and Cause-Specific Mortality and Life Expectancy in U.S. Adults', *Nutrients*, 13(8). ncbi.nlm.nih.gov/pmc/articles/PMC8401409/

84 Guarneiri, L.L. and Cooper, J.A. (2021) 'Intake of nuts or nut products does not lead to weight gain, independent of dietary substitution instructions: a systematic review and meta-analysis of randomized trials,' *Advances in Nutrition*, 12(2), pp. 384–401. doi.org/10.1093/advances/nmaa113

85 Basu, A., Devaraj, S. and Jialal, I. (2006) 'Dietary factors that promote or retard inflammation,' *Arteriosclerosis, Thrombosis, and Vascular Biology*, 26(5), pp. 995–1001. doi.org/10.1161/01.atv.0000214295.86079.d1

86 Beauchamp, G.K. et al. (2005) 'Ibuprofen-like activity in extra-virgin olive oil,' *Nature*, 437(7055), pp. 45–46. doi.org/10.1038/437045a

87 Guasch-Ferré, M. et al. (2022) 'Consumption of olive oil and risk of total and cause-wpecific mortality among U.S. adults,' *Journal of the American College of Cardiology*, 79(2), pp. 101–112. doi.org/10.1016/j.jacc.2021.10.041

88 Pes, G.M. et al. (2014) 'Male longevity in Sardinia, a review of historical sources supporting a causal link with dietary factors,' *European Journal of Clinical Nutrition*, 69(4), pp. 411–418. doi.org/10.1038/ejcn.2014.230

89 Maoloni, A. et al. (2020) 'Microbiological characterization of Gioddu, an Italian fermented milk,' *International Journal of Food Microbiology*, 323, p. 108610. doi.org/10.1016/j.ijfoodmicro.2020.108610

90 Brick, T. et al. (2016) 'ω-3 fatty acids contribute to the asthma-protective effect of unprocessed cow's milk,' *Journal of Allergy and Clinical Immunology*, 137(6), pp. 1699-1706.e13. doi.org/10.1016/j.jaci.2015.10.042

91 Societa' Agricola Casu'e Babbu S.S. (2023) Formaggi latte crudo non pastorizzato, Lodè, Nuoro. Casu'e Babbu casuebabbu.it/formaggio-con-latte-crudo/

92 Coelho, M.C., Malcata, F.X. and Silva, C. (2022) 'Lactic acid bacteria in Raw-Milk cheeses: From starter cultures to probiotic functions,' *Foods*, 11(15), p. 2276. doi.org/10.3390/foods11152276

93 EurekAlert. (2022) 'British toddlers and children consume too much added sugar, study suggests'. eurekalert.org

94 Blue Zones. (2023) Food guidelines. bluezones.com

95 Suez, J. et al. (2022) 'Personalized microbiome-driven effects of non-nutritive sweeteners on human glucose tolerance,' *Cell*, 185(18), pp. 3307-3328.e19. doi.org/10.1016/j.cell.2022.07.016

96 UCI MIND (2023) The 90+ Study –UCI MIND. mind.uci.edu/research-studies/90plus-study/

97 Kotifani, A. (2022) 'Longevity Link: How wine helps you live longer,' Blue Zones, 26 September. bluezones.com/2017/08/longevity-link-how-and-why-wine-helps-you-live-longer/

98 Haseeb, S., Alexander, B. and Baranchuk, A. (2017) 'Wine and cardiovascular health,' *Circulation*, 136(15), pp. 1434–1448. doi.org/10.1161/circulationaha.117.030387

99 Roy, C. et al. (2020) 'Red wine consumption associated with increased gut microbiota A-Diversity in 3 independent cohorts,' Gastroenterology, 158(1), pp. 270-272.e2. doi.org/10.1053/j.gastro.2019.08.024

100 Moreno-Indias, I. et al. (2016) 'Red wine polyphenols modulate fecal microbiota and reduce markers of the metabolic syndrome in obese patients,' Food & Function, 7(4), pp. 1775–1787. doi.org/10.1039/c5fo00886g

101 Droste, D.W. et al. (2013) 'A daily glass of red wine associated with lifestyle changes independently improves blood lipids in patients with carotid arteriosclerosis: results from a randomized controlled trial,' Nutrition Journal, 12(1). doi.org/10.1186/1475-2891-12-147

102 Jackson, R.S. (2020) 'Wine, food, and health,' in Elsevier eBooks, pp. 947–978. doi.org/10.1016/b978-0-12-816118-0.00012-x

103 Flanagan, E.W. et al. (2020) 'Calorie restriction and aging in humans,' *Annual Review of Nutrition*, 40(1), pp. 105–133. doi.org/10.1146/annurev-nutr-122319-034601

104 Mattison, J.A. et al. (2017) 'Caloric restriction improves health and survival of

rhesus monkeys,' *Nature Communications*, 8(1). doi.org/10.1038/ncomms14063.

105 Financial Times. Live long and prosper (June 21, 2013) ft.com/content

106 Nieddu, A. et al. (2020) 'Dietary habits, anthropometric features and daily performance in two independent long-lived populations from Nicoya peninsula (Costa Rica) and Ogliastra (Sardinia),' *Nutrients*, 12(6), p. 1621. doi.org/10.3390/nu12061621

107 Brandhorst, S. et al. (2024) 'Fasting-mimicking diet causes hepatic and blood markers changes indicating reduced biological age and disease risk,' *Nature Communications*, 15(1). doi.org/10.1038/s41467-024-45260-9

108 Acosta-Rodríguez, V.A. et al. (2022) 'Circadian alignment of early onset caloric restriction promotes longevity in male C57BL/6J mice,' *Science*, 376(6598), pp. 1192–1202. doi.org/10.1126/science.abk0297

109 King's College London (2023) '14-hour fasting improves hunger, mood and sleep,' King's College London, 14 November. kcl.ac.uk/news/14-hour-fasting-improves-hunger-mood-sleep.

110 Hurtado-Barroso, S. et al. (2019) 'Acute effect of a single dose of tomato sofrito on plasmatic inflammatory biomarkers in healthy men,' *Nutrients*, 11(4), p. 851. doi.org/10.3390/nu11040851

111 Shishehbor, F., Mansoori, A. and Shirani, F. (2017) 'Vinegar consumption can attenuate postprandial glucose and insulin responses; a systematic review and meta-analysis of clinical trials,' *Diabetes Research and Clinical Practice*, 127, pp. 1–9. doi.org/10.1016/j.diabres.2017.01.021

112 Novotny, J.A., Gebauer, S.K. and Baer, D.J. (2012) 'Discrepancy between the Atwater factor predicted and empirically measured energy values of almonds in human diets,' *The American Journal of Clinical Nutrition*, 96(2), pp. 296–301. doi.org/10.3945/ajcn.112.035782

113 Elizabeth, L. et al. (2020b) 'Ultra-Processed Foods and Health Outcomes: A Narrative review,' *Nutrients*, 12(7), p. 1955. doi.org/10.3390/nu12071955

114 National Food Strategy. (2021) The report - National Food Strategy. Nationalfoodstrategy.org

115 Gallagher, B.J. (2019) 'Ultra-processed foods make you eat more', BBC News, 16 May. bbc.co.uk/news/health-48280772

116 Hall, K.D. et al. (2019) 'Ultra-Processed diets cause excess calorie intake and weight gain: an inpatient randomized controlled trial of ad libitum food intake,' *Cell Metabolism*, 30(1), pp. 67-77.e3. doi.org/10.1016/j.cmet.2019.05.008

117 Tulleken, V.C. (2023) *Ultra processed people*. London: Penguin Random House.

118 Song, Z. et al. (2023) 'Effects of ultra-processed foods on the microbiota-gut-brain axis: The bread-and-butter issue,' *Food Research International*, 167.

119 BBC. (2021) What happened when I ate ultra-processed food for a month. bbc.co.uk/food/articles

120 Dalenberg, J.R. et al. (2020) 'Short-term consumption of sucralose with, but not without, carbohydrate impairs neural and metabolic sensitivity to sugar in humans,' *Cell Metabolism*, 31(3), pp. 493-502.e7. doi.org/10.1016/j.cmet.2020.01.014

121 Veldhuizen, M.G. et al. (2017) 'Integration of sweet taste and metabolism determines carbohydrate reward,' *Current Biology*, 27(16), pp. 2476-2485.e6. doi.org/10.1016/j.cub.2017.07.018

122 Tulleken, V.C. (2023) *Ultra processed people*. London: Penguin Random House.

123 Schatzker, M. (2022) *The end of craving*. Avid Reader Press / Simon & Schuster.

124 Shreiner, A.B., Kao, J.Y. and Young, V.B. (2015) 'The gut microbiome in health and in disease,' *Current Opinion in Gastroenterology*, 31(1), pp. 69–75. doi.org/10.1097/mog.0000000000000139

125 David, L.A. et al. (2013) 'Diet rapidly and reproducibly alters the human gut microbiome,' *Nature*, 505(7484), pp. 559–563. doi.org/10.1038/nature12820

126 U.S. Department of Agriculture. (2018) FoodData Central fdc.nal.usda.gov

127 Çatalkaya, G. et al. (2020) 'Interaction of dietary polyphenols and gut microbiota: Microbial metabolism of polyphenols, influence on the gut microbiota, and implications on host health,' Food Frontiers, 1(2), pp. 109–133. doi.org/10.1002/fft2.25.

128 Plamada, D. and Vodnar, D.C. (2021) 'Polyphenols – gut microbiota interrelationship: a transition to a new generation of prebiotics,' *Nutrients*, 14(1), p. 137. doi.org/10.3390/nu14010137

129 Massy, H. (2023) 10 best foods/drinks that are high in polyphenols | ZOE. zoe.com/learn/foods-high-in-polyphenols.

130 McDonald, D. et al. (2018) 'American gut: an open platform for citizen science microbiome research,' MSystems, 3(3). doi.org/10.1128/msystems.00031-18

131 Stanford Medicine. (2021) 'Fermented-food diet increases microbiome diversi-

ty, decreases inflammatory proteins, study finds', med.stanford.edu/

132 Lozupone, C. et al. (2012) 'Diversity, stability and resilience of the human gut microbiota,' *Nature*, 489(7415), pp. 220–230. doi.org/10.1038/nature11550

133 Wastyk H.C., Fragiadiakis G.K., Perelman D et al. (2021) 'Gut-microbiota-targeted diets modulate human immune status', *Cell*, 184(16) pp.4137-4153 https://www.cell.com/cell/fulltext/S0092-8674(21)00754-6

134 Jacka, F.N. et al. (2017) 'A randomised controlled trial of dietary improvement for adults with major depression (the "SMILES" trial),' *BMC Medicine*, 15(1). doi.org/10.1186/s12916-017-0791-y

135 Food and mood centre. (2019) 'The SMILEs Trial' foodandmoodcentre.com.au

136 Bridges, F. (2019) 'Healthy food makes you happy: Research shows a healthy diet improves your mental health,' *Forbes*, 26 January. forbes.com

137 Mujcic, R. and Oswald, A.J. (2016) 'Evolution of well-being and happiness after increases in consumption of fruit and vegetables,' *American Journal of Public Health*, 106(8), pp. 1504–1510. doi.org/10.2105/ajph.2016.303260

138 Harbec, M.-J. and Pagani, L.S. (2018) 'Associations between early family meal environment quality and later Well-Being in School-Age children,' *Journal of Developmental and Behavioral Pediatrics*, 39(2), pp. 136–143. doi.org/10.1097/dbp.0000000000000520

139 Berge, J.M. et al. (2015) 'The protective role of family meals for youth obesity: 10-Year Longitudinal Associations,' *The Journal of Pediatrics*, 166(2), pp. 296–301. doi.org/10.1016/j.jpeds.2014.08.030

140 Walton, K. et al. (2018) 'Exploring the role of family functioning in the association between frequency of family dinners and dietary intake among adolescents and young adults,' *JAMA Network Open*, 1(7), p. e185217. doi.org/10.1001/jamanetworkopen.2018.5217

141 Walton, K. et al. (2018) 'Exploring the role of family functioning in the association between frequency of family dinners and dietary intake among adolescents and young adults,' *JAMA Network Open*, 1(7), p. e185217. doi.org/10.1001/jamanetworkopen.2018.5217

142 Behie, A.M. and Pavelka, M.S.M. (2012) 'The role of minerals in food selection in a black howler monkey (Alouatta pigra) population in Belize following a major hurricane,' *American Journal of Primatology*, 74(11), pp. 1054–1063. doi.org/10.1002/ajp.22059

143 Davis, C.M. (1928) 'Self selection of diet by newly weaned infants',

American Journal of Diseases of Children, 36(4). doi.org/10.1001/archpedi.1928.01920280002001

144 Davis, C.M. (1939) Results of self-selection of diets by young children, pubmed.ncbi.nlm.nih.gov/20321464/

145 Alcock, J., Maley, C.C. and Aktipis, A. (2014) 'Is eating behavior manipulated by the gastrointestinal microbiota? Evolutionary pressures and potential mechanisms,' *BioEssays*, 36(10), pp. 940–949. doi.org/10.1002/bies.201400071

146 Wolpert, S. (2019) 'Dieting does not work, UCLA researchers report,' UCLA, 10 May. newsroom.ucla.edu

147 Lowe, M.R. et al. (2013) 'Dieting and restrained eating as prospective predictors of weight gain,' *Frontiers in Psychology*, 4. doi.org/10.3389/fpsyg.2013.00577

Index

advertising, processed foods 119, 121
ageing *see also* longevity
  chronological and biological 138–9
alcohol 94–7
almonds 72, 110, 124
Alzheimer's disease 80
Amati, Frederica 61–2, 91–2
amino acids 61–2, 70, 109, 128
anchovies
  broccoli and anchovy pasta 168
  mozzarella with anchovies, lemon and parsley 182
appetite *see also* satiety
  brain 37–8
  hormone signals 70, 115–16
  nutritional intelligence 133–8
artichokes 124
artichokes with parsley and hazelnuts 180
artificial sweeteners 93–4, 119–20
asparagus
  asparagus, tarragon and Parmesan risotto 172–3
  spring vegetable minestrone 176–7
aspartame 94
astringency 133
Athena 75–6
Atkins, Robert 45
aubergine parmigiana 186–7

bacteria *see* fermentation; gut microbiome
Banting, William 44
barley
  root vegetable soup with barley 212
  soluble fibre 47
beans
  borlotti bean, squash and chard stew 224–5
  broadbeans and ricotta on sourdough 166
  butterbean and mushroom stew with chestnuts and thyme 208–9
  cannellini beans with chicken, sage and tomatoes 189–90
  chilli and garlic greens and beans 196–7
  fish soup 181–2
  green beans in tomato sauce 185
  Italy 11–12
  pasta e fagioli 204–5
  protein 60
  spring vegetable minestrone 176–7
beef
  mushroomy bolognese 202–3
  slow-cooked beef with thyme, garlic and brown lentils 230–1
beetroot 97
  mackerel with pickled beetroot 195
belonging, sense of 18
Berry, Sarah 109
beta-glucan 47
blackberry and orange olive oil pudding 211
blood pressure: nitric oxide 97
blood sugar levels
  insulin resistance 91
  legumes 70
  monitoring 92–3
  sourdough bread 47
  vinegar 79
blue zones
  carbohydrates 43, 46–7, 48
  dairy products 81–5
  eating together 17, 130, 156
  exercise 42, 141–2
  first identification 13–15
  introduction of processed foods 120–1

legumes 67
meat 54–6, 62
not overeating 103, 109
nuts 72
olive oil 76
overview of way of life 17–18, 159–62
plant based diets 49–53
protein 43
social networks 140–1
sugar 89–90
wine 94
blueberries 52
borlotti bean, squash and chard stew 224–5
brain
  ageing and diet 48
  appetite 37–8
bread
  broadbeans and ricotta on sourdough 166
  creamed chard on toast 183
  Italy 12
  Sardinia 43, 46–7
  sourdough 47–8, 160
breakfast cereals 89
broadbeans
  broadbeans and ricotta on sourdough 166
  spring vegetable minestrone 176–7
broccoli and anchovy pasta 168
Brunstrom, Jeff 135, 136
Buettner, Dan 15, 56, 95
Burt, Hattie 118
butterbeans
  butterbean and mushroom stew with chestnuts and thyme 208–9
  pasta e fagioli 204–5
butternut squash see squash

cabbage and pecorino gratin 170–1
California: Loma Linda 15, 49, 50–1, 67, 72, 76, 141–2
Calment, Jeanne Louise 17
calorie restriction 101–3
calories
  counting 110
  not all equal 75, 111–12
cancer
  alcohol 94–5
  aspartame 94
  dairy products 82
  fasting 105
  meat 57, 58, 63–4
  nuts 73
  olive oil 80
  sugar 91
  ultra-processed foods (UPFs) 32
cannellini beans
  cannellini beans with chicken, sage and tomatoes 189–90
  chilli and garlic greens and beans 196–7
  spring vegetable minestrone 176–7
capers
  cannellini beans with chicken, sage and tomatoes 189–90
  fish soup 181–2
  sardines with tomatoes, capers, lemon and basil 188
  warm potato salad with capers, dill and lemon 177
caraway and chilli braised baby gem 200–1
carbohydrates
  blue zones 43, 46–7, 48
  caloric availability 112
  complex 45–6
  refined 46
  simple 45–6
carcinogens 63–4
cardiovascular health *see also* cholesterol
  fibre 124
  nuts 74
  olive oil 80–1

sugar 91
ultra-processed foods (UPFs) 32
wine 97
carrots
  best chicken stock 228–9
  borlotti bean, squash and chard stew 224–5
  mirepoix/soffritto 109–10
  mushroomy bolognese 202–3
  New Year's Day lentil soup 219–20
  pasta e fagioli 204–5
  root vegetable soup with barley 212
  slow-cooked beef with thyme, garlic and brown lentils 230–1
  spring vegetable minestrone 176–7
Caruso, Salvatore 65, 106–7
cauliflower: caramelised cauliflower, onion and garlic dip 218
cavolo nero
  chilli and garlic greens and beans 196–7
  New Year's Day lentil soup 219–20
Cecchini, Dario 71–2
Celea, Vincenza 65–6, 103, 142–3
celeriac: root vegetable soup with barley 212
celery
  best chicken stock 228–9
  borlotti bean, squash and chard stew 224–5
  mirepoix/soffritto 109–10
  mushroomy bolognese 202–3
  New Year's Day lentil soup 219–20
  pasta e fagioli 204–5
  root vegetable soup with barley 212
  slow-cooked beef with thyme, garlic and brown lentils 230–1
  spring vegetable minestrone 176–7
watercress and basil soup with toasted walnuts 167
centenarians 13–14, 15–16, 48, 130
chard
  borlotti bean, squash and chard stew 224–5
  creamed chard on toast 183
cheese
  asparagus, tarragon and Parmesan risotto 172–3
  aubergine parmigiana 186–7
  bitter leaf salad with burrata, pears and walnuts 216
  broadbeans and ricotta on sour dough 166
  cabbage and pecorino gratin 170–1
  chickpea, feta and dill filo pie 198–9
  mozzarella with anchovies, lemon and parsley 182
  pasta e fagioli 204–5
  pumpkin fritters with salsa verde 214–15
  radicchio, orange and feta salad with toasted walnuts 169
  raw milk 84
  ricotta with figs, nuts and honey 205
  Sardinia 83, 84, 85
chestnuts 124
  butterbean and mushroom stew with chestnuts and thyme 208–9
chicken
  best chicken stock 228–9
  cannellini beans with chicken, sage and tomatoes 189–90
  mushroom broth with chicken and garlic 222–3
  protein 60
  soup, benefit of 114
  used as seasoning 54–6
chickpeas

chickpea, feta and dill filo pie
    198–9
chickpeas with clams, garlic and
    parsley 178–9
hummus 69
chicory 124
  bitter leaf salad with burrata,
    pears and walnuts 216
  chicory with herbs, chilli and
    lemon 221
chilli and garlic greens and beans
    196–7
children
  eating together 130–1
  height 36
  nutritional intelligence 134–5
  obesity 30–1
  raw milk 84
  school lunches 31–2
  sugar consumption levels 89
chilli and garlic greens and beans
    196–7
chocolate 124
cholesterol 24, 47, 70, 96
Chrysohoou, Christina 103
clams: chickpeas with clams, garlic
    and parsley 178–9
coeliac disease 30
coffee 51–2, 133
cold water exposure 143
comfort food 126
community, sense of 18, 140–1
Contaldo, Gennaro 147–9
convenience food 23–4, 34–5, 151
  see also ultra-processed foods
cooking
  benefits of 19–20, 113–14,
    161–2
  happiest diet 150–3
cost of food 34, 35, 150–1, 154
Costa Rica *see* Nicoya
courgettes
  fried courgette with white wine
    vinegar and mint 193
  spring vegetable minestrone
    176–7
cravings: nutritional intelligence
    135–6
creativity 143
Crete 75
cucina povera 146–9

dairy products *see also* cheese; milk;
    yoghurt
  blue zones 81–5
  nutrition 27
  pasteurisation 84, 85
Davis, Clara 134–5
dementia 63, 80, 107
depression: Mediterranean diet
    127
desserts see puddings
diabetes *see also* blood sugar levels
  artificial sweeteners 93–4
  Banting diet 44
  dementia 107
  fibre 124
  ultra-processed foods (UPFs) 32
diaita 157, 158, 159–62
diet *see also* blue zones; fasting;
    nutrition
  calorie-counting 110
  diversification 138
  effect on health and ageing
    18–19, 20–1
  low-carb 44–5
  low-fat 24–6
  Mediterranean 26, 57–8, 96, 127
  not 'dieting' 157–8
  plant based 49–53
  social media tribalism 27–8
  way of life 157, 158, 159–62
diet culture 29–30
Dimbleby, Henry 31
disease, diet-related 31, 34
Dunbar, Robin 131–2

eating together 17, 129–32, 155–6
eggs
  onion and herb frittata 217

protein 60
endorphins 131–3
environment, obesogenic 38–9
exercise, natural 17, 42, 141–2, 144

fast food undernourishment 35–6
fasting 101–3, 104–6, 108–9
fat, dietary *see also* olive oil
  blue zones 43
  caloric availability 112
  historical advice against 24–6
  longevity 80–1
feeding windows 108–9
fennel: white wine braised fennel 210
fermentation
  dairy products 82–5
  gut microbiome 125
  sourdough bread 47
feta: chickpea, feta and dill filo pie 198–9
fibre
  barley 47
  caloric availability 112
  gut microbiome 123–4
  legumes 69, 123–4
  mental health 127
  recommended intake 123–4
  soluble 47
fight or flight mode 142, 143
figs: ricotta with figs, nuts and honey 205
fish
  blue zones 51
  broccoli and anchovy pasta 168
  fish soup 181–2
  mackerel with pickled beetroot 195
  mozzarella with anchovies, lemon and parsley 182
  protein 60
  sardines with tomatoes, capers, lemon and basil 188
flavour and food choices

blue zones 40–1
calories not all equal 112–13
happiest diet 145–9
olive oil 78–9, 80
food accessibility
  costs 34, 35
  obesogenic environments 38–9
Food Foundation 34, 35
food processing: NOVA classification 32–3
Frasconi, Pasquale 13
fregola salad with herbs 191
friendships 18, 95, 131–3, 139–40

genes
  compared to lifestyle factors 14–15
  obesity 36–7, 38–9
Global Burden of Disease study 18–19
glucose *see* blood sugar levels
gluten 29–30, 47
grape juice concentrate 118–19
Greece *see also* Ikaria
  mythology of olive oil 75–6
green beans in tomato sauce 185
Guasch-Ferre, Marta 81
gut microbiome
  artificial sweeteners 93–4
  blue zones 121
  diversification 138
  evolution 123
  fermented foods 125
  fibre 70, 123–4
  gut–brain axis 128
  mental health 127
  plant based diet 124
  polyphenols 73, 79
  prebiotics 83
  probiotics 83
  resveratrol 96
  second brain 121–2, 137–8
  size 121
  ultra-processed foods (UPFs) 117
gym culture 59

Hall, Kevin 114
happiness 125–6, 128, 131–2
haricot beans: fish soup 181–2
hazelnuts 124
  artichokes with parsley and hazelnuts 180
health span 16
hedonic region, brain 38
Heggie, Lisa 89
height, nutritional effects on 36
herbs 51
Hippocrates 76
Homer 75
honey
  ricotta with figs, nuts and honey 205
  strawberries with honeyed nuts, thyme and lemon 194
  thyme and lemon poached pears 226–7
Hook, Steve 84
hummus 69
hunger
  brain and genes 37–8
  hormone signals 115–16
Hyman, Mark 56
hypothalamus 37

Ikaria, Greece
  dairy products 85
  first identified as blue zone 15
  herbal tea 97
  legumes 67
  meat 54
  not overeating 103
  olive oil 76
  plant based diet 49, 51
  wine 95
ikigai 18, 141
India 12
inflammation 73, 79, 91–2, 105, 139–40
ingredient labels 33, 34, 118–19
instincts 40
insulin resistance 91–2

intuitive eating 133–8
Irish Longitudinal Study on Ageing (TILDA) 138–9
Italy *see also* Sardinia
  cucina povera 146–9
  gluten 30
  legumes 67–8
  Molochio, Calabria 65–7, 100–1, 102–3, 106–7
  typical diets 10, 11–12

Jacka, Felice 126–7
Japan *see also* Okinawa *ikigai* 18, 141

kale: orzo with squash and kale 206–7
Kawas, Claudia 95
kefir 83
Kenny, Rose Anne 138–40, 141, 142, 143, 144
'keto' diets 44
khichdi 12

lactic acid 47
lactose-intolerance 84
lamb 54
  slow-cooked leg of lamb with crispy potatoes 174–5
leeks
  best chicken stock 228–9
  butterbean and mushroom stew with chestnuts and thyme 208–9
  cannellini beans with chicken, sage and tomatoes 189–90
  slow-cooked leeks with lemon and walnuts 213
  spring vegetable minestrone 176–7
Leeming, Emily 122, 128
legumes 66–72, 123–4 *see also* beans
lemons
  chickpea, feta and dill filo pie

198–9
chicory with herbs, chilli and lemon 221
mozzarella with anchovies, lemon and parsley 182
sardines with tomatoes, capers, lemon and basil 188
slow-cooked leeks with lemon and walnuts 213
strawberries with honeyed nuts, thyme and lemon 194
thyme and lemon poached pears 226–7
warm potato salad with capers, dill and lemon 177

lentils
 fibre 124
 New Year's Day lentil soup 219–20
 slow-cooked beef with thyme, garlic and brown lentils 230–1
lettuce: caraway and chilli braised baby gem 200–1
Li, Yanping 74
Lo Franco, Bandino 79–80, 81
Loma Linda, California 15, 49, 50–1, 67, 72, 76, 141–2
loneliness 139–40
longevity
 alcohol 95
 blue zones 13–18
 fasting 101–3, 104–6
 legumes 68
 nuts 73–4
 olive oil 80–1
Longo, Assunta 143
Longo, Valter 65, 99–100, 102, 104–7
lycopene 109, 110
lysine 70

mackerel with pickled beetroot 195
maltodextrins 117
mangiafoglie 11

Matarozzo, Angelo 103, 143–4
Mazzei, Francesco 80, 155
McCay, Clive 101–2
meat
 ageing and consumption levels 62–3
 blue zones 54–6
 nutrition and health 56–9
 processed foods 63–4
 quality 64
 used as seasoning 54–6, 64
 Western consumption 56
MEDAS questionnaire 58, 96
Mediterranean diet 26, 57–8, 96, 127
Mele, Gianni 85
mental health 125–8, 139–40
microbiome *see* gut microbiome
milk
 non-dairy 23–4
 nutrition 26–7
 quality 82
 raw 84–5
mindfulness 20, 143
minestrone 49, 55
 spring vegetable minestrone 176–7
mirepoix 109–10
modified starch 25, 116–17
Molochio, Calabria, Italy 65–7, 100–1, 102–3, 106–7
Monteiro, Carlos 32
mood and food 125–8
Mosley, Michael 60
mozzarella
 aubergine parmigiana 186–7
 mozzarella with anchovies, lemon and parsley 182
mushrooms
 butterbean and mushroom stew with chestnuts and thyme 208–9
 mushroom broth with chicken and garlic 222–3
 mushroomy bolognese 202–3

mussels: fish soup 181–2

New Year's Day lentil soup 219–20
Nicoya, Costa Rica
  first identified as blue zone 15
  legumes 67
  meat 62
  not overeating 103
  nuts 72
  plant based diet 49, 50
  sense of purpose 141
  'three sisters' 109
nitrates 97
Non-Communicable Diseases Risk Factor Collaboration 36
NOVA classification 32–3
nutrition *see also* diet
  dairy products 27
  effects on height 36
  fasting 104–5
  food combinations 109–10
  legumes 68–71
  meat 56–9
  nitrates 97
  nuts 73–5
  olive oil 79–80
  plant based diets 49–50
  'protein package' 61
  wine with meals 96, 97
nutritional intelligence 133–8
nutritional mismatch 119–20, 136–7
nuts
  artichokes with parsley and hazel nuts 180
  bitter leaf salad with burrata, pears and walnuts 216
  calories 110
  definition 72–3
  dietary fat 26
  nutrition 73–5, 124
  radicchio, orange and feta salad with toasted walnuts 169
  ricotta with figs, nuts and honey 205
  slow-cooked leeks with lemon and walnuts 213
  strawberries with honeyed nuts, thyme and lemon 194
  watercress and basil soup with toasted walnuts 167

oat milk 24
obesity 30–1, 36–7, 38–9, 137
Okinawa, Japan
  first identified as blue zone 15
  legumes 67
  meat 54
  not overeating 103
  plant based diet 50, 61
  sweet potato 48
  wine 95
Okinawan Ratio 48
oleic acid 79
olive oil 26, 75–81, 124
  blackberry and orange olive oil pudding 211
  food combinations and nutrients 109
omega-3s 84
onions
  best chicken stock 228–9
  borlotti bean, squash and chard stew 224–5
  caramelised cauliflower, onion and garlic dip 218
  mirepoix/soffritto 109–10
  onion and herb frittata 217
  pasta e fagioli 204–5
  peperonata 197
  polyphenols 124
  root vegetable soup with barley 212
  slow-cooked beef with thyme, garlic and brown lentils 230–1
oranges
  blackberry and orange olive oil pudding 211
  radicchio, orange and feta salad with toasted walnuts 169

orzo with squash and kale 206–7
overeating
  not 17, 103, 161
  ultra-processed foods (UPFs) 114–15, 117–18
Ozempic 70

pancetta: mushroomy bolognese 202–3
Parkinson's disease 80
parsnips: root vegetable soup with barley 212
pasta
  broccoli and anchovy pasta 168
  fregola salad with herbs 191
  fresh tomato spaghetti 192–3
  mushroomy bolognese 202–3
  orzo with squash and kale 206–7
  pasta e fagioli 67–8, 204–5
  spring vegetable minestrone 176–7
pasteurisation 84, 85
pears
  bitter leaf salad with burrata, pears and walnuts 216
  thyme and lemon poached pears 226–7
peas with mustard and dill 184
pecans 124
  strawberries with honeyed nuts, thyme and lemon 194
peperonata 197
peppers: peperonata 197
Peretti, G. 43
Pes, Gianni 13, 15
pie, chickpea, feta and dill filo 198–9
pistachios 72
  ricotta with figs, nuts and honey 205
plant based diets
  blue zones 49–53
  legumes 66–72
  nuts 72–5
  ultra-processed foods (UPFs) 53–4
polyphenols
  blueberries 52
  food combinations 110
  gut microbiome 79
  legumes 124
  nuts 73, 124
  olive oil 79, 124
  olive water 81
  wine 95, 96, 97, 124
pork 54
  mushroomy bolognese 202–3
Poseidon 76
potatoes 50
  slow-cooked leg of lamb with crispy potatoes 174–5
  warm potato salad with capers, dill and lemon 177
  watercress and basil soup with toasted walnuts 167
prebiotics 83
Predimed study 58
probiotics 83
processed foods 31–5, 53, 112, 151
protein
  amino acids 61–2, 70
  blue zones 43
  caloric availability 112
  daily requirements 60
  function in the body 59–60
  legumes 70
  meat 56, 59
  nutritional mismatch 119–20
  plant sources 61–2
  protein products 59
'protein leverage hypothesis' 60
'protein package' 61
puddings
  blackberry and orange olive oil pudding 211
  ricotta with figs, nuts and honey 205
  strawberries with honeyed nuts, thyme and lemon 194

thyme and lemon poached pears 226–7
pulses 67
pumpkin fritters with salsa verde 214–15
purpose, sense of 18, 141

radicchio
  bitter leaf salad with burrata, pears and walnuts 216
  radicchio, orange and feta salad with toasted walnuts 169
ratatouille 12
Raubenheimer, David 60
Rauber, Fernanda 33
resveratrol 96
rice: asparagus, tarragon and Parmesan risotto 172–3
ricotta
  broadbeans and ricotta on sourdough 166
  ricotta with figs, nuts and honey 205
Romans, ancient 76
Romeo, Domenico 65
root vegetable soup with barley 212

salads
  bitter leaf salad with burrata, pears and walnuts 216
  fregola salad with herbs 191
  radicchio, orange and feta salad with toasted walnuts 169
  sardines with tomatoes, capers, lemon and basil 188
  warm potato salad with capers, dill and lemon 177
sardines with tomatoes, capers, lemon and basil 188
Sardinia
  bread 42–3, 46–7
  dairy products 82–4
  exercise 141
  first identified as blue zone 13–14
  legumes 67
  meat 55, 62
  olive oil 76
  plant based diet 49–50
  wine 95
satiety *see also* overeating
  beta-glucan 47
  hormone signals 70, 115–16
  legumes 69, 70
  nuts 75
Schatzker, Mark 119–20, 135, 136
seafood
  chickpeas with clams, garlic and parsley 178–9
  fish soup 181–2
seasonal eating 12, 153–5
self-control 37
serotonin 128
Seventh-Day Adventists 50–1, 72, 141–2
sex life satisfaction 143
Shannon, Oliver 57, 59, 97
Simpson Steve 60
sleep 143
Small, Dana 119–20
social eating 17, 129–32, 155–6
social media 27
social networks 17, 18, 95, 131–2, 139–40
soffritto 109–10
Sonnenburg, Justin 125
soups
  benefit of chicken soup 114
  fish soup 181–2
  minestrone 49
  mushroom broth with chicken and garlic 222–3
  New Year's Day lentil soup 219–20
  nutrition 49
  root vegetable soup with barley 212
  spring vegetable minestrone 176–7

watercress and basil soup with toasted walnuts 167
sourdough bread 160
Spector, Tim 26–7
spices 133
spring vegetable minestrone 176–7
squash
  borlotti bean, squash and chard stew 224–5
  orzo with squash and kale 206–7
  pumpkin fritters with salsa verde 214–15
starch, modified 25, 116–17
strawberries with honeyed nuts, thyme and lemon 194
stress reduction 18, 142–3
sugar *see also* blood sugar levels
  blue zones 89–90
  consumption levels 88–9
  grape juice concentrate 118–19
  health effects 91–2
  low-fat yoghurts 25
  processed foods 87–8, 90
  puddings and celebrations 85–7, 89–90
'superfoods' 42, 52, 74
Suzuki, Makoto 15
sweet potato 48
sweeteners, artificial 93–4, 119–20

tannins 133
tea 96–7, 133
TILDA (Irish Longitudinal Study on Ageing) 138–9
tofu 124
tomatoes 10–11
  added sugar 87–8
  aubergine parmigiana 186–7
  best chicken stock 228–9
  borlotti bean, squash and chard stew 224–5
  cannellini beans with chicken, sage and tomatoes 189–90
  fish soup 181–2
  fresh tomato spaghetti 192–3
  green beans in tomato sauce 185
  lycopene 109, 110
  mozzarella with anchovies, lemon and parsley 182
  mushroomy bolognese 202–3
  New Year's Day lentil soup 219–20
  peperonata 197
  sardines with tomatoes, capers, lemon and basil 188
  sofritto 79
  spring vegetable minestrone 176–7
Trimarchi, Giovanna 102–3, 149
tryptophan 128

UK
  children's height 36
  health span 16
  obesity 30–1
  ultra-processed foods (UPFs) consumption 114
ultra-processed foods (UPFs) 31–5, 53–4, 112, 113–21, 151, 152
umami 54

van Tulleken, Chris 116–18, 120
vegetables
  Italy 12
  plant based diets 49–53
vinegar 79

walnuts 73
  bitter leaf salad with burrata, pears and walnuts 216
  radicchio, orange and feta salad with toasted walnuts 169
  slow-cooked leeks with lemon and walnuts 213
  strawberries with honeyed nuts, thyme and lemon 194
  watercress and basil soup with toasted walnuts 167
  watercress and basil soup with

  toasted walnuts 167
weight loss
  beta-glucan 47
  diet culture 29–30
  eating real food 159
  legumes 69, 70
  low-carb diets 44–5
  nuts 75
  obesogenic environments 39
  Ozempic 70
Williams, Liz 34, 82
willpower 37
wine 17, 94–7, 124
Wren, Gavin 27–8

yeast 104
Yeo, Giles 36–7, 38, 111–12
yoghurt
  added sugar 89
  blue zones 82–3, 85, 125
  low-fat 23, 24, 25
  strawberries with honeyed nuts,
    thyme and lemon 194

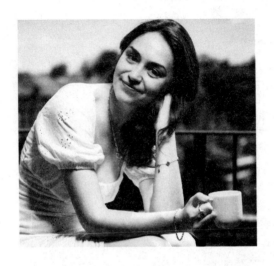

Giulia Crouch writes on food and health for national newspapers including the *Times*, the *Mail* and the *Sun*, and is co-host of a weekly food segment on Times Radio. She lives in London, but still makes regular visits to her family's homes in Sardinia and southern Italy.